OUTLIVE LONGEVITY COOKBOOK AND FITNESS PLAN

Inspired by Dr. Peter Attia's Approach - A Science-Backed Nutrition and Exercise Blueprint for Lifelong Strength and Vitality

TOMMY B. ATTIA

Copyright

MEDICAL DISCLAIMER

The content in this book is for informational and educational purposes only. It is not intended as a substitute for professional medical advice, diagnosis, or treatment. Always seek the advice of your physician or other qualified health provider with any questions you may have regarding a medical condition, fitness program, or nutritional plan.

Never disregard professional medical advice or delay in seeking it because of something you have read in this book. The author and publisher are not responsible for any adverse effects or consequences resulting from the use of any suggestions, preparations, or procedures described in this book.

Before beginning any new exercise program or making significant changes to your diet, consult with a healthcare professional, especially if you have existing health conditions, are taking medications, or have a history of heart disease, high blood pressure, diabetes, or other chronic conditions.

The exercise programs and nutritional recommendations in this book are not intended for individuals with specific medical limitations unless approved by a physician. Individual results may vary based on starting fitness level, adherence to the program, genetic factors, and overall health status.

If you experience pain, dizziness, shortness of breath, or any unusual symptoms during exercise, stop immediately and consult a healthcare provider.

The author and publisher disclaim any liability for any injury, loss, or damage incurred as a consequence, directly or indirectly, of the use and application of any of the contents of this book.

To every person who chose to begin again.

To those who train not for vanity, but for the decades ahead.

To anyone who has ever said: "I want to feel strong at seventy."

This book is for you.

FOREWORD

There is a quiet revolution happening in how we think about aging.

For generations, we accepted decline as inevitable. We watched our parents slow down, lose strength, and struggle with tasks that were once simple. We assumed this was the natural order of things, the unavoidable consequence of getting older.

But the science tells a different story.

We now know that much of what we call aging is not aging at all. It is disuse. It is metabolic dysfunction. It is the accumulated result of thousands of small decisions, habits, and environmental inputs that either support or erode our capacity.

The truth is both sobering and empowering: the body you will inhabit at seventy is being built today. Not by luck. Not by genetics alone. But by what you eat, how you move, how you sleep, and how you recover.

This book is not a quick fix. It is not a thirty-day transformation or a miracle protocol. It is something far more valuable: a sustainable system for building and maintaining the physical capacity that allows you to live fully, independently, and powerfully for as long as possible.

The approach you will find here is inspired by the emerging field of Medicine 3.0, a paradigm that prioritizes prevention over intervention and healthspan over lifespan. It focuses not on adding years to life, but on adding life to years. It asks not just how long you will live, but how well you will live.

This book synthesizes evidence-based principles from exercise science, metabolic health, and nutritional biochemistry into a practical framework that anyone can follow. It is designed for people who want clarity, not complexity. Who want systems, not fads. Who understand that longevity is not a single decision but a daily practice.

You will learn how to eat in a way that stabilizes blood sugar, preserves muscle, and supports energy without dogma or restriction. You will discover how to train your body not just for today, but for the demands of the next three, four, or five decades. You will understand why recovery is not optional, and how sleep and stress management are as critical as any workout or meal.

Most importantly, you will learn that it is never too late to start. Whether you are thirty or seventy, active or sedentary, strong or struggling, the principles in this book can meet you where you are and move you forward.

The goal is not perfection. It is progress. Not intensity, but consistency. Not deprivation, but awareness. Not youth, but vitality.

This is your invitation to train for the long game. To build a body that serves you not just now, but for all the years to come.

Let's begin.

Table of Contents

INTRODUCTION

Longevity Isn't Luck — It's Practice

There is a photograph that sits on my desk. It shows a woman in her late seventies, smiling as she hoists a grocery bag in each hand. She is walking up a flight of stairs without holding the railing. Her posture is upright. Her stride is confident. She is not frail. She is not dependent. She is capable.

This woman is not an outlier. She is not genetically blessed. She is not wealthy or particularly fortunate. What she is, quite simply, is prepared.

For decades, she moved her body intentionally. She ate to support her metabolism, not to punish herself. She prioritized sleep. She managed stress. She built muscle when it was still easy to build, and she maintained it when it became harder. She understood something that many people do not: the body you will inhabit in your later years is being shaped right now, by what you do today.

This is the central premise of longevity science, and it is both humbling and hopeful. We cannot control everything about how we age, but we can control far more than we think. The question is not whether aging will happen. It will. The question is whether we will age with strength, independence, and vitality, or whether we will age with frailty, dependency, and disease.

For most of human history, we had no choice. Aging meant decline. Medicine focused on treating diseases after they appeared, not on preventing them. Fitness was for athletes, not for everyday people trying to live well into their eighties. Nutrition was about avoiding deficiency, not optimizing metabolism.

But the landscape has shifted. We now have decades of research showing that many of the conditions we associate with aging, such as sarcopenia, insulin resistance, cardiovascular disease, and cognitive decline, are not inevitable. They are often the result of modifiable behaviors. They are, in many cases, preventable.

This is the promise of what some researchers call Medicine 3.0, a new paradigm that shifts focus from reactive treatment to proactive optimization. Instead of waiting for disease to appear and then managing it, we ask a different question: what can we do now to extend not just lifespan, but healthspan, the period of life in which we are fully functional, energetic, and free from chronic illness?

The answer is neither mysterious nor complicated. It comes down to three interconnected pillars: how we move, how we eat, and how we recover. These are not separate domains. They are synergistic. Movement drives metabolic health. Nutrition supports movement and recovery. Recovery enables consistent movement. Together, they form a sustainable system for building and maintaining the physical capacity that defines a long, healthy life.

Yet despite the clarity of the science, most people struggle to apply it. Not because they lack willpower or discipline, but because they lack a framework. They are drowning in conflicting advice. They have been told to eat less and move more, but they do not know what that actually means in practice. They have tried diets that promise transformation but deliver only temporary results and long-term frustration. They have started exercise programs that were too intense, too boring, or too disconnected from their real-world needs.

1

This book is designed to solve that problem. It is not a collection of tips or hacks. It is a comprehensive, evidence-based system for longevity that integrates nutrition, fitness, and recovery into a single, cohesive plan. It is designed for real people with real lives, people who want to be strong and capable at seventy, not just thin at forty. People who understand that health is not a project with an end date, but a practice that evolves over a lifetime.

The approach you will find here is grounded in science but written for clarity. It does not require you to count every calorie, track every macro, or spend hours in the gym. It does not demand perfection. It demands consistency. It asks you to make small, sustainable changes that compound over time, building a foundation of strength, metabolic health, and resilience that will serve you for decades.

Let me be clear about what this book is not. It is not a quick fix. It will not promise you a six-pack in six weeks or a miracle transformation in thirty days. Those promises are seductive, but they are also short-sighted. They focus on aesthetics, not function. They prioritize speed over sustainability. They measure success in pounds lost, not in capacity gained.

This book takes a different view. It measures success not by how you look in a mirror, but by what you can do. Can you lift your grandchildren without straining your back? Can you hike for miles without exhaustion? Can you stand up from the floor without using your hands? Can you carry your groceries, climb stairs, travel independently, and live without fear of falling or injury?

These are the metrics that matter. These are the markers of a life well-lived. And they are entirely within your control.

The foundation of this approach is muscle. Not because muscle makes you look better, although it often does, but because muscle is the organ of longevity. It is metabolic tissue that regulates blood sugar, supports bone density, protects joints, and preserves independence. When you lose muscle, you lose capacity. You become weaker, slower, more fragile. You increase your risk of falls, fractures, and metabolic disease. You lose the ability to do the things you love.

This process, called sarcopenia, begins as early as your thirties if you do nothing to prevent it. But here is the good news: it is preventable. With consistent resistance training, adequate protein intake, and proper recovery, you can not only stop muscle loss but reverse it. You can build strength at fifty, sixty, seventy, and beyond. You can become more capable, not less, as you age.

The second pillar is metabolic health. Your metabolism is not just about weight. It is about how efficiently your body processes energy, how stable your blood sugar remains, how well your cells respond to insulin, and how effectively you use the food you eat. Poor metabolic health leads to insulin resistance, type 2 diabetes, cardiovascular disease, and cognitive decline. Good metabolic health supports energy, longevity, and resilience.

Nutrition plays a central role here, but not in the way most diet books suggest. This is not about eliminating food groups or following rigid meal plans. It is about understanding how food affects your body and making choices that support stable blood sugar, preserve muscle, and provide sustained energy. It is about eating real food, prioritizing protein, managing carbohydrate intake based on activity level, and avoiding the blood sugar rollercoaster that drives hunger, fatigue, and disease.

The third pillar is recovery. This is the most overlooked component of longevity, yet it is just as important as movement and nutrition. Recovery is not passive. It is not about doing nothing. It is about creating the conditions that allow your body to adapt, repair, and grow stronger. Sleep is the cornerstone of recovery, influencing everything from hormone regulation to immune function to cognitive performance. Stress management is equally critical, as chronic stress disrupts metabolism, impairs recovery, and accelerates aging.

These three pillars, movement, nutrition, and recovery, form the foundation of the system you will learn in this book. They are not isolated strategies. They are integrated practices that reinforce one another. When you train consistently, you improve insulin sensitivity, which makes your nutrition more effective. When you eat to support muscle and energy, you recover better, which allows you to train harder. When you prioritize sleep and manage stress, you enhance both metabolic health and physical performance.

This is the feedback loop of longevity. Every positive choice makes the next one easier. Every small improvement compounds into something larger. Over weeks, months, and years, these practices transform not just your body, but your relationship with aging itself.

The structure of this book reflects this integrated approach. Part I lays the conceptual foundation, explaining what longevity really means and why traditional approaches to health and fitness often fall short. You will learn how metabolism works, why muscle matters, and what it means to train for decades, not just for today.

Part II focuses on nutrition, providing clear principles for eating in a way that supports metabolic health and muscle preservation without dogma or restriction. You will learn how to build meals that stabilize blood sugar, when to eat more or less based on activity, and how to stock a kitchen that makes healthy eating effortless. This section includes fifty-five recipes designed specifically for longevity, each one tested, practical, and aligned with the metabolic principles you will learn.

Part III presents the Longevity Fitness Plan, a twelve-week progressive training program that builds strength, cardiovascular capacity, stability, and mobility. The program is designed for real people at any starting point, whether you are returning to exercise after years of inactivity or looking to optimize an existing routine. It is structured in phases that build on one another, creating a sustainable system you can follow for life.

Part IV addresses recovery, exploring the science of sleep, stress, and hormonal health. You will learn practical strategies for improving sleep quality, managing stress, and supporting the recovery processes that make all your other efforts effective.

Part V ties everything together, showing you how to live this system in the real world. You will learn how to track progress without obsession, how to adjust the plan as your life changes, and how to build consistency without perfection. This is where philosophy meets practice, where the knowledge becomes habit, and where longevity becomes identity.

One of the questions I am asked most often is: when should I start? The answer is always the same: now. Whether you are thirty or seventy, whether you have never exercised or have been training for years, the principles in this book can meet you where you are and move you forward. The science is clear: it is never too early to build capacity, and it is never too late to improve.

If you are young, this book will teach you how to build a foundation that will serve you for decades. You will learn habits that prevent the decline most people accept as inevitable. You will invest in your future self.

If you are middle-aged, this book will show you how to reverse the early signs of metabolic dysfunction and muscle loss. You will regain strength, energy, and confidence. You will redefine what aging looks like.

If you are older, this book will prove that decline is not destiny. You will learn that you can still build muscle, improve mobility, and enhance your quality of life. You will discover that capability is not about age, but about practice.

This is not a book you read once and put on a shelf. It is a manual you return to, a system you refine, a practice you live. The recipes will feed you. The workouts will challenge you. The recovery strategies will restore you. And over time, all of it will transform you.

But transformation is not the goal. Capacity is. The goal is to be strong enough to live the life you want, for as long as possible. To travel without exhaustion. To play with your grandchildren without pain. To remain independent, capable, and vital well into your later years.

The goal is to age with dignity, strength, and joy. To look at the person in the photograph, the one carrying groceries up the stairs with a smile, and to recognize yourself.

That future is not determined by luck. It is built by practice. And the practice begins now.

This introduction has set the foundation for everything that follows. You now understand that longevity is not about living longer at any cost, but about living better for as long as possible. You know that the body you will inhabit in your later years is being shaped today by the choices you make around movement, nutrition, and recovery.

As you move through this book, you will encounter specific strategies, detailed workouts, and tested recipes. But never lose sight of the bigger picture: these are tools for building capacity. They are practices that compound over time. They are investments in your future self.

Before you continue to Chapter 1, take a moment to reflect on your own relationship with aging.

What does longevity mean to you?

What do you want to be able to do at seventy, eighty, or beyond?

What fears do you have about losing capacity, and what hopes do you have for maintaining it?

Write these thoughts down. Keep them close. They will remind you why you started when the work becomes difficult. They will anchor you to your purpose when motivation fades. They will guide you back to practice when life pulls you away.

Longevity is not luck. It is practice. And your practice begins now.

CHAPTER 1: RETHINKING LONGEVITY

We have been asking the wrong question.

For decades, the focus of medicine, public health, and personal wellness has been on a single metric: how long can we live? We measure success in years added, diseases delayed, and mortality rates reduced. We celebrate breakthroughs that extend lifespan, and we fear anything that might shorten it.

But longevity, in its truest sense, is not about the number of years you accumulate. It is about the quality of life you maintain within those years. It is about the difference between existing and living, between surviving and thriving, between dependency and autonomy.

Consider two people, both of whom live to eighty-five. The first spends their final fifteen years in and out of hospitals, managing multiple chronic conditions, relying on others for basic tasks, and experiencing a steady erosion of physical and cognitive function. The second remains active, independent, and engaged until the very end, experiencing a brief period of decline only in their final months.

Both lived to eighty-five. But they did not live the same life.

This distinction is the heart of modern longevity science, and it is where we must begin if we are to understand what we are truly optimizing for.

Lifespan vs Healthspan

The terms sound similar, but they represent fundamentally different goals.

Lifespan is simple. It is the total number of years you live from birth to death. It is the number on your tombstone. For most of human history, increasing lifespan was the primary goal of medicine. We focused on preventing early death from infectious disease, trauma, and acute illness. We succeeded remarkably well. Life expectancy in developed countries has more than doubled in the past century.

But somewhere along the way, we discovered a troubling truth: adding years to life does not necessarily add life to years.

Healthspan is different. It is the period of your life during which you are healthy, functional, and free from chronic disease and disability. It is the years you can move without pain, think clearly, live independently, and do the things that bring you joy. It is not measured in calendar years, but in capacity.

The gap between lifespan and healthspan is where suffering lives. It is the years spent in decline, the decade or more of managing multiple medications, the slow loss of independence, the inability to do the things you once took for granted. For many people, this gap spans ten, fifteen, or even twenty years. They are alive, but they are not living well.

The goal of modern longevity science is to compress this gap, to extend healthspan so that it matches lifespan as closely as possible. The aim is not to live to one hundred in a state of frailty and dependence, but to live to ninety or one hundred with full function, experiencing only a brief period of decline at the very end.

This is called compression of morbidity, and it is entirely achievable. The science is clear: most of what we call aging is not inevitable biological decay. It is the accumulated result of choices, behaviors, and environmental factors that either support or erode our capacity.

The question is not whether you will age. You will. The question is how you will age. Will you age with strength, mobility, and independence? Or will you age with frailty, pain, and dependence? The difference is largely within your control.

The Four Horsemen of Chronic Disease

If we want to extend healthspan, we need to understand what shortens it. The answer is not mysterious. Four categories of chronic disease account for the vast majority of suffering, disability, and premature death in the developed world. These are sometimes called the four horsemen: cardiovascular disease, cancer, neurodegenerative disease, and metabolic dysfunction.

Cardiovascular disease includes heart attacks, strokes, and heart failure. It remains the leading cause of death globally. The underlying process, atherosclerosis, begins decades before symptoms appear. Plaque builds up in the arteries, narrowing blood flow and increasing the risk of clots. By the time you experience chest pain or have a heart attack, the disease is already advanced.

Cancer is the second horseman. It is not a single disease, but hundreds of different diseases that share a common feature: uncontrolled cell growth. Some cancers are highly influenced by genetics, but many are driven by modifiable factors such as smoking, obesity, chronic inflammation, and metabolic dysfunction.

Neurodegenerative disease includes Alzheimer's, Parkinson's, and other conditions that erode cognitive and motor function. These diseases are devastating not just because they shorten life, but because they rob people of their identity, memory, and independence long before death.

Metabolic dysfunction is the fourth horseman, and it is the most insidious because it underlies the other three. This category includes insulin resistance, type 2 diabetes, obesity, and non-alcoholic fatty liver disease. Metabolic dysfunction does not just cause suffering on its own. It accelerates cardiovascular disease, increases cancer risk, and contributes to neurodegeneration.

Here is what matters: these diseases are not inevitable. They are not simply the result of bad genes or bad luck. They are largely the result of modifiable behaviors. The way you eat, the way you move, the way you sleep, and the way you manage stress all influence your risk for each of these conditions.

Traditional medicine waits for these diseases to appear and then treats them. A longevity-focused approach asks a different question: what can we do now to prevent these diseases from ever taking hold?

The answer lies in building and maintaining the physical and metabolic capacity that protects against them. This is not about adding one more drug or supplement. It is about foundational practices that support health at a cellular level.

Why Strength and Metabolism Matter More Than Scale Weight

If you have spent any time thinking about health or fitness, you have almost certainly stepped on a scale and judged yourself by the number you saw. This is what we have been taught to do. Weight is the metric we track, the number we compare, the goal we set.

But weight is a terrible indicator of health.

Two people can weigh the same and have completely different body compositions, completely different metabolic health, and completely different functional capacities. One might be lean and muscular with excellent insulin sensitivity and strong bones. The other might be metabolically unhealthy with low muscle mass, high body fat, and poor physical function. The scale cannot tell the difference.

What matters is not your weight. It is your body composition, your metabolic health, and your physical capacity.

Muscle is the organ of longevity. It is metabolically active tissue that burns calories at rest, regulates blood sugar, supports bone density, protects joints, and preserves independence. When you have adequate muscle mass, your body is more resilient. You recover faster from illness. You maintain your metabolism. You stay strong enough to do the things that matter.

When you lose muscle, everything gets harder. Your metabolism slows. Your blood sugar becomes less stable. Your bones weaken. Your risk of falls and fractures increases. Your independence erodes.

Muscle loss with aging, called sarcopenia, is one of the most significant threats to healthspan. It begins as early as your thirties and accelerates after fifty if you do nothing to prevent it. The average person loses three to eight percent of their muscle mass per decade after thirty, with the rate increasing after sixty.

But here is the critical point: this loss is not inevitable. It is preventable and, in many cases, reversible. Resistance training, combined with adequate protein intake, can build muscle at any age. Studies show that even people in their eighties and nineties can gain significant strength and muscle mass with proper training.

Metabolic health is equally important. Your metabolism is not just about weight. It is about how efficiently your body processes energy, how stable your blood sugar remains, how well your cells respond to insulin, and how effectively you use the food you eat.

Poor metabolic health is at the root of most chronic disease. Insulin resistance, the hallmark of metabolic dysfunction, drives type 2 diabetes, cardiovascular disease, fatty liver disease, and even some cancers and neurodegenerative conditions. It is not benign. It is not just about being overweight. It is a systemic problem that affects every organ in your body.

Good metabolic health, on the other hand, is protective. It supports energy, resilience, and longevity. It allows your body to use food efficiently, maintain stable blood sugar, and avoid the inflammatory cascade that drives disease.

The scale cannot measure muscle mass. It cannot measure metabolic health. It cannot measure strength, function, or capacity. It gives you a number that means almost nothing in the context of longevity.

What you should care about instead is: How much muscle do I have? How strong am I? How stable is my blood sugar? How well does my body respond to insulin? Can I lift, carry, climb, and move without pain? Can I recover quickly from exertion? These are the metrics that matter.

This shift in focus changes everything. It changes what you eat, how you train, and what you measure. It moves you away from restriction and toward building. It moves you away from obsessing over pounds lost and toward celebrating capacity gained.

You are not trying to weigh less. You are trying to be stronger, more metabolically healthy, and more capable. The scale is irrelevant. The work is what matters.

Aging as a Performance Problem, Not Just Decline

We have been conditioned to think of aging as a process of inevitable decline. We watch older adults slow down, lose strength, and struggle with tasks that were once simple, and we assume this is just what happens. We accept it as natural, unavoidable, and beyond our control.

But what if aging is not primarily a biological problem? What if it is a performance problem?

Consider an athlete who stops training. Within weeks, their cardiovascular fitness declines. Within months, they lose muscle mass and strength. Within a year, they are a shadow of their former selves. This is not aging. This is deconditioning. It is the result of removing the stimulus that maintained their capacity.

Now consider the average adult. They graduate from school and become less active. They get a desk job and spend most of their day sitting. They stop playing sports. They stop lifting heavy things. They stop moving in varied, challenging ways. Their body adapts to this new reality by becoming weaker, less mobile, and less resilient.

Decades pass. They are now sixty, and they have lost significant muscle mass, bone density, cardiovascular fitness, and joint mobility. They assume this is aging. But it is not. It is the cumulative effect of decades of insufficient stimulus.

The body adapts to the demands placed on it. If you demand nothing, it gives you nothing. If you demand strength, it builds strength. If you demand endurance, it builds endurance. If you demand stability and mobility, it maintains them.

This is the principle of adaptation, and it does not stop at any age. Your body remains responsive to training stimulus throughout your entire life. The rate of adaptation may slow, but it does not disappear. You can build muscle at seventy. You can improve cardiovascular fitness at eighty. You can enhance mobility and balance at ninety.

This reframe is powerful. It means that aging is not something that happens to you. It is something that happens in response to how you live. If you live in a way that preserves capacity, you will age differently than someone who does not.

Think of aging as a performance curve. Everyone starts at a certain level of capacity in their twenties or thirties. From there, the curve can take different trajectories. One person maintains a high level of capacity well into their seventies and eighties, experiencing only a brief, steep decline at the very end. Another person experiences a slow, steady decline starting in their forties, losing capacity gradually over decades until they are frail and dependent long before they die.

The difference between these two trajectories is not genetics, although genetics play a role. The difference is behavior. It is the cumulative effect of thousands of small decisions about how to move, what to eat, how to sleep, and how to recover.

If you train consistently, you maintain muscle and strength. If you eat to support your metabolism, you avoid insulin resistance and metabolic dysfunction. If you prioritize sleep, you allow your body to recover and adapt. If you manage stress, you protect your hormonal balance and immune function.

These practices do not stop the aging process. They shape it. They determine whether you age with capability or with frailty. They determine whether you remain independent or become dependent. They determine the quality of your final decades.

This is the mindset that guides everything in this book. Aging is not a disease to be cured. It is a process to be optimized. It is not something that happens to you. It is something you participate in. And the choices you make today, every single day, are shaping the body and mind you will inhabit for the rest of your life.

You cannot control your genes. You cannot control your chronological age. But you can control your biological age, your functional capacity, and your healthspan. You can decide whether you will age like someone who trains or like someone who does not.

The difference is profound. And the time to start is now.

This chapter has established the foundational principles that will guide everything else in this book. You now understand that longevity is not about adding years to life, but about adding life to years. You know the difference between lifespan and healthspan, and you understand that the goal is to compress the gap between them.

You have been introduced to the four horsemen of chronic disease: cardiovascular disease, cancer, neurodegenerative disease, and metabolic dysfunction. These are not inevitable. They are largely preventable through the choices you make about movement, nutrition, sleep, and stress.

You now know that weight is not the metric that matters. What matters is muscle mass, metabolic health, and functional capacity. You are not trying to weigh less. You are trying to be stronger, healthier, and more capable.

Finally, you have learned to reframe aging as a performance problem rather than an inevitable decline. Your body adapts to the demands you place on it. If you train it, feed it, and recover it properly, you can maintain extraordinary capacity well into your later years.

Before moving to Chapter 2, take a moment to reflect on how you currently think about aging. Do you see it as inevitable decline, or as something you can influence? What fears do you have about losing capacity, and what hopes do you have for maintaining it?

Write these thoughts down. They will serve as a reference point as you build the practices that will shape your healthspan.

Aging is not something that happens to you. It is something you participate in. And your participation begins with awareness, intention, and action.

CHAPTER 2: METABOLISM MADE PRACTICAL

If you have ever felt confused about metabolism, you are not alone.

The word gets thrown around constantly in diet books, fitness magazines, and wellness blogs, usually accompanied by promises to "boost" it, "fix" it, or "hack" it. But most of these explanations are either oversimplified to the point of being useless or overcomplicated to the point of being inaccessible.

The truth is that metabolism is not a single thing you can speed up or slow down with a magic food or supplement. It is a vast, interconnected network of chemical processes that govern how your body converts food into energy, builds and repairs tissue, regulates hormones, and maintains every function necessary for life.

But while metabolism is complex, the principles that matter for longevity are not. You do not need a PhD in biochemistry to understand how your metabolism works or what you can do to optimize it. You just need clarity on a few key concepts.

In this chapter, we will cut through the noise and focus on what actually matters: blood sugar stability, insulin sensitivity, muscle as a metabolic organ, protein requirements as you age, and the balance between inflammation and recovery. These are the levers you can control. These are the factors that determine whether your metabolism supports longevity or undermines it.

Let's start with the foundation.

Blood Sugar Stability (No Obsession)

Your body runs on fuel, and the primary fuel it uses is glucose, a simple sugar that circulates in your bloodstream. Every cell in your body, particularly your brain and muscles, relies on a steady supply of glucose to function.

When you eat, especially when you eat carbohydrates, your blood sugar rises. This is normal and expected. Your body releases insulin, a hormone produced by the pancreas, to move that glucose out of your bloodstream and into your cells where it can be used for energy or stored for later use.

After your cells take up the glucose they need, your blood sugar drops back down to a baseline level. This rise and fall is a natural rhythm that happens multiple times a day. The key question is: how dramatic is that rise and fall?

If your blood sugar rises moderately and returns to baseline smoothly, you feel stable. Your energy is consistent. Your hunger is manageable. Your mood is even. Your body handles the glucose efficiently, and your cells remain responsive to insulin.

But if your blood sugar spikes sharply and crashes quickly, you feel it. You get a burst of energy followed by fatigue. You feel hungry again soon after eating. You might feel irritable, foggy, or anxious. Your body has to release large amounts of insulin to manage the spike, and over time, this pattern creates problems.

Chronic blood sugar instability is not just uncomfortable. It is metabolically damaging. When your blood sugar spikes repeatedly, your cells are exposed to high levels of glucose, which is inflammatory and toxic at high concentrations. Your pancreas has to work overtime to produce insulin. Your cells, constantly bombarded with insulin, begin to lose their sensitivity to it. This is the beginning of insulin resistance, the root cause of metabolic dysfunction.

The goal is not to eliminate blood sugar fluctuations. That is neither possible nor desirable. The goal is to keep those fluctuations within a healthy range so that your body can manage them efficiently without stress or damage.

This is what we mean by blood sugar stability. It is not about obsessively tracking your glucose levels with a continuous monitor, although some people find that useful. It is about eating in a way that produces moderate, manageable blood sugar responses rather than extreme spikes and crashes.

How do you do this? The answer is simpler than you might think.

First, prioritize protein and fat at every meal. Both macronutrients slow the absorption of carbohydrates, blunting the blood sugar spike. A meal with protein, fat, and carbohydrates will produce a much gentler blood sugar curve than a meal with carbohydrates alone.

Second, choose carbohydrates that are less refined and higher in fiber. Whole grains, legumes, vegetables, and fruits produce smaller blood sugar responses than white bread, pasta, pastries, and sugary snacks. Fiber slows digestion, which slows glucose absorption.

Third, eat carbohydrates in the context of activity. Your muscles are glucose sinks. When you exercise, especially when you do resistance training or high-intensity work, your muscles become more sensitive to insulin and better at taking up glucose. Eating carbohydrates after training supports recovery and produces a smaller blood sugar spike than eating the same carbohydrates while sedentary.

Fourth, avoid grazing. Eating small amounts of food constantly keeps your blood sugar and insulin elevated all day. Eating structured meals with gaps in between allows your blood sugar and insulin to return to baseline, giving your cells a break from constant stimulation.

These are not rigid rules. They are principles. You do not need to follow them perfectly. You just need to follow them consistently enough that your blood sugar remains mostly stable most of the time.

This is the foundation of metabolic health. Everything else builds on this.

Insulin Sensitivity Explained Simply

Insulin is one of the most important hormones in your body, yet most people do not understand what it does or why it matters.

Think of insulin as a key that unlocks your cells so glucose can enter. When you eat and your blood sugar rises, your pancreas releases insulin into your bloodstream. Insulin travels to your cells and binds to receptors on their surface, signaling them to open up and allow glucose inside.

When this system works well, your cells respond quickly to insulin. They open up, take in the glucose they need, and your blood sugar returns to normal. This is called insulin sensitivity, and it is a good thing. It means your body is efficient at managing blood sugar with minimal insulin.

But when this system stops working well, your cells become less responsive to insulin. They do not open up as easily. Your pancreas has to release more and more insulin to get the same effect. This is called insulin resistance, and it is the root of metabolic dysfunction.

Insulin resistance does not happen overnight. It develops gradually over years or even decades. At first, your pancreas compensates by producing more insulin. Your blood sugar stays normal, but your insulin levels are elevated. You feel fine. You have no symptoms. But behind the scenes, damage is accumulating.

Eventually, your pancreas cannot keep up. It cannot produce enough insulin to overcome the resistance. Your blood sugar starts to rise. You develop prediabetes, then type 2 diabetes. By this point, you have likely had insulin resistance for a decade or more.

But the damage is not limited to blood sugar. Chronically elevated insulin has widespread effects. It promotes fat storage, particularly around the abdomen. It increases inflammation. It contributes to high blood pressure and cardiovascular disease. It is associated with certain cancers and neurodegenerative diseases. Insulin resistance is not just a diabetes problem. It is a whole-body problem.

The good news is that insulin sensitivity is highly responsive to lifestyle interventions. You can improve it, often dramatically, with the right strategies.

Exercise is the most powerful tool. When you exercise, particularly when you do resistance training or high-intensity interval work, your muscles become more sensitive to insulin. They take up glucose more efficiently, even without much insulin present. This effect lasts for hours or even days after your workout.

Losing excess body fat, particularly visceral fat around the abdomen, also improves insulin sensitivity. Visceral fat is metabolically active and produces inflammatory signals that contribute to insulin resistance. Reducing it has a direct, positive effect on metabolic health.

Eating to support stable blood sugar, as discussed in the previous section, reduces the demand for insulin in the first place. When you avoid constant blood sugar spikes, your pancreas does not have to work as hard, and your cells are not constantly exposed to high insulin levels.

Sleep and stress management also play a role. Poor sleep and chronic stress both impair insulin sensitivity through hormonal pathways we will discuss in later chapters. Prioritizing rest and recovery is not optional if you want to maintain metabolic health.

Here is the key point: insulin sensitivity is not fixed. It is dynamic. It changes based on what you do. If you are currently insulin resistant, you are not stuck. You can reverse it. If you are currently insulin sensitive, you can maintain or improve it. The levers are in your hands.

Insulin sensitivity is one of the most important markers of metabolic health and longevity. When your cells respond well to insulin, everything works better. Your energy is stable. Your body composition improves. Your risk of chronic disease drops. You feel better, perform better, and age better.

This is why metabolic health is foundational to everything else in this book. You cannot build a body that lasts if your metabolism is broken.

Muscle as a Metabolic Organ

When most people think about muscle, they think about strength, appearance, or athletic performance. But muscle is far more than a tool for lifting weights or looking good. It is a metabolic organ, one of the most important in your body.

Muscle is metabolically active tissue. Unlike fat, which is relatively inert, muscle burns calories even at rest. The more muscle you have, the higher your resting metabolic rate. This is one reason why people with more muscle mass tend to maintain a healthy weight more easily than people with less muscle.

But muscle's metabolic role goes far beyond calorie burning. Muscle is the primary site of glucose disposal in the body. When you eat carbohydrates, most of that glucose is taken up by your muscles, either to be used immediately for energy or to be stored as glycogen for later use.

This makes muscle your body's largest glucose sink. The more muscle you have, and the more you use it, the better your body is at managing blood sugar. Your muscles act as a buffer, absorbing glucose and preventing blood sugar spikes.

This is why resistance training is so powerful for metabolic health. When you train your muscles, you increase their size, their insulin sensitivity, and their capacity to store glycogen. You improve your body's ability to handle carbohydrates. You reduce your risk of insulin resistance and type 2 diabetes.

But the benefits extend beyond blood sugar management. Muscle produces signaling molecules called myokines when you contract it. These myokines have widespread effects throughout the body. They reduce inflammation. They support immune function. They improve brain health. They enhance fat metabolism. Muscle is not just a passive tissue. It is an endocrine organ that communicates with the rest of your body.

Muscle also supports bone density. When you load your muscles through resistance training, you create mechanical stress on your bones. Your bones respond by becoming denser and stronger. This is why people who lift weights have stronger bones than people who do only cardio or no exercise at all. The relationship between muscle and bone is bidirectional and mutually reinforcing.

Then there is the longevity factor. Muscle mass is one of the strongest predictors of healthy aging. Studies consistently show that people with more muscle mass live longer, have lower rates of chronic disease, and maintain independence later in life. Muscle is protective.

The flip side is equally important. Losing muscle, which begins in your thirties and accelerates after fifty if you do nothing to prevent it, has catastrophic consequences. As muscle declines, so does your metabolic health. Your resting metabolic rate drops. Your insulin sensitivity worsens. Your ability to handle carbohydrates declines. Your risk of type 2 diabetes, cardiovascular disease, and other chronic conditions increases.

Muscle loss also means functional decline. You become weaker. Everyday tasks become harder. Your risk of falls and fractures increases. Your independence erodes. Sarcopenia, the age-related loss of muscle mass, is not a cosmetic problem. It is a functional and metabolic crisis.

But here is the empowering part: you can prevent it. You can even reverse it. Muscle is highly responsive to training stimulus at any age. Even people in their eighties and nineties can build significant muscle mass with proper resistance training and adequate protein intake.

This is why strength training is non-negotiable for longevity. It is not optional. It is not just for athletes or bodybuilders. It is for anyone who wants to maintain metabolic health, physical function, and independence as they age.

You are not training to look like a fitness model. You are training to preserve the organ that regulates your metabolism, protects your bones, and maintains your capacity to live fully.

Muscle is metabolic insurance. Build it while you can. Maintain it as long as you can. Your future self will thank you.

Why Protein Matters More as We Age

Protein is the most important macronutrient for longevity, yet it is the one most people under-consume, especially as they age.

Protein is made up of amino acids, the building blocks your body uses to build and repair tissue. Your muscles, bones, skin, hair, enzymes, hormones, and immune cells are all made of protein. Every day, your body breaks down and rebuilds proteins in a constant cycle of turnover. To maintain this process, you need a steady supply of dietary protein.

When you are young, your body is highly efficient at using protein. You can build and maintain muscle relatively easily, even with modest protein intake. But as you age, this changes. Your body becomes less efficient at processing protein. This is called anabolic resistance.

Anabolic resistance means that your muscles do not respond as strongly to the signal to build and repair. You need more protein, and more of the essential amino acid leucine in particular, to stimulate the same muscle protein synthesis response that you got with less protein when you were younger.

If you do not increase your protein intake as you age, you lose muscle. This is one of the primary drivers of sarcopenia. The typical diet, which is often heavy on carbohydrates and light on protein, simply does not provide enough amino acids to prevent muscle loss in older adults.

But when you increase protein intake, especially in combination with resistance training, you can prevent muscle loss and even build new muscle. The research is clear: older adults who consume higher amounts of protein maintain more muscle mass, more strength, and better physical function than those who consume less.

How much protein do you need? The current recommended dietary allowance, which is 0.8 grams per kilogram of body weight per day, is widely considered inadequate for active older adults. Most longevity-focused experts recommend significantly more.

A reasonable target for adults over forty who are training regularly is approximately 1.6 to 2.2 grams of protein per kilogram of body weight per day, or roughly 0.7 to 1.0 grams per pound. For a 150-pound person, this translates to about 105 to 150 grams of protein per day.

This might sound like a lot if you are not used to tracking protein, but it is achievable with intentional meal planning. Each meal should contain a substantial protein source: eggs, Greek yogurt, or protein powder at breakfast; chicken, fish, or legumes at lunch; beef, pork, or tofu at dinner. Snacks can include protein-rich options like cottage cheese, nuts, or protein shakes.

Protein distribution also matters. Rather than consuming most of your protein at one meal, aim to spread it across three or four meals. Each meal should contain at least 25 to 40 grams of protein to maximally stimulate muscle protein synthesis. This pattern is more effective for building and maintaining muscle than eating small amounts of protein throughout the day or loading it all into one meal.

Leucine, one of the essential amino acids, is particularly important. It is the primary trigger for muscle protein synthesis. Animal proteins like meat, poultry, fish, eggs, and dairy are rich in leucine. Plant proteins tend to be lower in leucine, which is why vegetarians and vegans often need to consume more total protein to achieve the same muscle-building effect.

This is not a criticism of plant-based diets. It is simply a recognition that protein quality and amino acid composition matter. If you eat a plant-based diet, you can absolutely meet your protein needs, but you need to be more intentional about it. Combining different plant protein sources, consuming higher total protein, and possibly supplementing with essential amino acids can help bridge the gap.

Beyond building muscle, protein has other benefits for longevity. It is highly satiating, meaning it keeps you full longer and reduces overall calorie intake without conscious restriction. It has a higher thermic effect than carbohydrates or fats, meaning your body burns more calories digesting and processing it. It supports immune function, hormone production, and tissue repair throughout your body.

Protein is not just for bodybuilders. It is for anyone who wants to maintain muscle, metabolic health, and physical function as they age. It is one of the simplest, most powerful tools you have for building a body that lasts.

If you take one nutritional action from this chapter, make it this: increase your protein intake. Track it for a week to see where you currently stand. Then adjust your meals to hit your target consistently. The difference it makes over months and years is profound.

Inflammation vs Recovery Balance

Inflammation is one of the most misunderstood concepts in health and fitness. It has become a buzzword, blamed for everything from weight gain to chronic disease to aging itself. And while chronic inflammation is indeed problematic, inflammation itself is not the enemy. It is a necessary part of how your body responds to stress, injury, and infection.

The key is balance.

There are two types of inflammation: acute and chronic. Acute inflammation is the immediate response to injury or infection. When you cut your finger, twist your ankle, or catch a cold, your immune system sends white blood cells and inflammatory signals to the affected area. This is a good thing. It is how your body repairs damage and fights off pathogens. Acute inflammation is temporary, targeted, and essential for healing.

Chronic inflammation is different. It is low-grade, persistent, and systemic. It is not triggered by a specific injury or infection. Instead, it is the result of ongoing stressors such as poor diet, lack of exercise, insufficient sleep, chronic stress, obesity, or environmental toxins. Chronic inflammation does not heal. It damages.

Over time, chronic inflammation contributes to insulin resistance, cardiovascular disease, neurodegenerative disease, and cancer. It accelerates aging at a cellular level. It is one of the hallmarks of metabolic dysfunction.

But here is where things get interesting: exercise creates inflammation. When you train, particularly when you do resistance training or high-intensity work, you create microscopic damage to your muscle fibers. This triggers an acute inflammatory response. Your body sends immune cells and inflammatory signals to the damaged tissue to begin the repair process.

This is not a problem. This is the process of adaptation. The inflammation caused by exercise is temporary, localized, and productive. It is what allows your muscles to rebuild stronger, your cardiovascular system to improve, and your metabolism to become more efficient.

The problem arises when the inflammatory stress from training exceeds your ability to recover. If you train too hard, too often, without adequate rest, nutrition, or sleep, the acute inflammation from exercise becomes chronic. Your body cannot keep up with the repair demands. You become overtrained, fatigued, and more susceptible to injury and illness.

This is why recovery is not optional. It is not a luxury for elite athletes. It is a fundamental part of the training process. Recovery is when adaptation happens. It is when your body repairs the damage from training, rebuilds tissue, and emerges stronger than before.

The balance between training stress and recovery capacity determines whether your training makes you healthier or sicker, stronger or weaker, more resilient or more fragile.

So how do you maintain this balance? The answer involves multiple factors, all of which we will explore in detail later in this book.

First, you need adequate nutrition. Your body cannot repair tissue without the raw materials to do so. Protein provides the amino acids for muscle repair. Carbohydrates replenish glycogen stores. Fats support hormone production and reduce inflammation. Micronutrients, particularly vitamins C, D, and E, along with minerals like zinc and magnesium, support immune function and recovery processes.

Second, you need sleep. This is non-negotiable. Sleep is when your body produces growth hormone, repairs tissue, clears metabolic waste from your brain, and regulates the hormones that control hunger, stress, and metabolism. Chronic sleep deprivation impairs recovery, increases inflammation, and undermines every other effort you make to improve your health.

Third, you need to manage training volume and intensity. More is not always better. There is a dose-response relationship with exercise. Too little, and you do not create enough stimulus for adaptation. Too much, and you exceed your recovery capacity. Finding the right dose requires awareness, honesty, and sometimes a willingness to do less.

Fourth, you need stress management. Psychological stress triggers the same inflammatory pathways as physical stress. If your life is chronically stressful, your body is in a constant state of inflammatory activation. This impairs recovery, disrupts sleep, and accelerates aging. Practices like breathwork, meditation, time in nature, and meaningful social connection all reduce stress and support recovery.

Finally, you need to listen to your body. Fatigue, persistent soreness, declining performance, poor sleep, increased resting heart rate, and frequent illness are all signs that your recovery is not keeping pace with your training. These are not signs of weakness. They are feedback. Ignoring them leads to breakdown.

The goal is not to eliminate inflammation. It is to create just enough inflammatory stress to drive adaptation, followed by enough recovery to allow that adaptation to occur. This is the balance that builds a body that lasts.

When you get this balance right, training makes you healthier. When you get it wrong, training breaks you down. The difference is recovery.

This chapter has taken you inside the engine of longevity: your metabolism. You now understand that metabolism is not a single thing to be "boosted" or "fixed," but a complex system that responds to how you live.

You have learned that blood sugar stability is foundational. Keeping your blood sugar within a healthy range, without obsessive tracking, protects you from insulin resistance and metabolic dysfunction. You do this by prioritizing protein and fat, choosing quality carbohydrates, timing carbohydrates around activity, and avoiding constant grazing.

You have learned that insulin sensitivity is not fixed. It is dynamic and highly responsive to exercise, body composition, nutrition, sleep, and stress management. Improving insulin sensitivity is one of the most powerful things you can do for your long-term health.

You now know that muscle is not just about strength or appearance. It is a metabolic organ that regulates blood sugar, produces beneficial signaling molecules, supports bone density, and predicts longevity. Building and maintaining muscle is non-negotiable.

You understand that protein requirements increase as you age due to anabolic resistance. Consuming adequate protein, distributed across multiple meals, is essential for maintaining muscle mass and metabolic health. This is one of the simplest, most impactful nutritional changes you can make.

Finally, you have learned that inflammation is not inherently bad. Acute inflammation from training is necessary for adaptation. The problem is chronic inflammation, which arises when training stress exceeds recovery capacity. The balance between stress and recovery determines whether your efforts build you up or break you down.

Before moving to Chapter 3, take a moment to assess your current metabolic health. Do you experience energy crashes after meals? Are you hungry shortly after eating? Do you carry excess body fat, particularly around your abdomen? Are you consuming enough protein? Are you balancing training stress with adequate recovery?

These questions will help you identify where to focus your efforts. Metabolic health is not built overnight, but every meal, every training session, and every night of sleep is an opportunity to move in the right direction.

Your metabolism is not your enemy. It is a system that responds to input. Give it the right input, and it will serve you for decades.

CHAPTER 3: TRAINING FOR THE LONG GAME

There is a fundamental difference between training for performance and training for longevity.

Performance training asks: how fast can I run? How much can I lift? How well can I compete? It is about pushing limits, chasing personal records, and maximizing output in a specific domain. It is intensive, specialized, and often unsustainable over decades.

Longevity training asks a different question: what physical capacities do I need to maintain independence, function, and vitality for the rest of my life? It is about building a broad base of strength, endurance, stability, and mobility that will serve you not just today, but when you are seventy, eighty, or ninety. It is about training in a way that is sustainable, joint-friendly, and progressive without being destructive.

Most people train as if they are preparing for a competition that will never come. They push hard, ignore pain, skip recovery, and wonder why they are injured, burnt out, or unable to maintain consistency. They confuse intensity with effectiveness. They mistake suffering for progress.

Longevity training requires a different mindset. It is not about how hard you can push today. It is about how well you can move for the next fifty years. It is not about maximal effort. It is about optimal effort, the minimum effective dose of training that produces adaptation without exceeding your capacity to recover.

This chapter will introduce you to the framework that makes longevity training possible. You will learn why strength is the foundation of everything else, how cardiovascular training supports metabolic health and resilience, why VO_2 max matters even if you never test it, how mobility and joint integrity preserve your ability to move, and why rest is not the opposite of training but an essential part of it.

Let's begin with the currency of longevity: strength.

Strength as Longevity Currency

If you could only do one type of training for the rest of your life, it should be resistance training. Nothing else comes close to the broad, systemic benefits that strength training provides.

Strength is not just about being able to lift heavy things, although that is part of it. Strength is about force production, the ability to generate enough muscular force to move your body and external objects through space. Every time you stand up from a chair, climb stairs, carry groceries, lift a suitcase, or catch yourself from falling, you are using strength.

As you age, strength becomes the limiting factor in almost everything you do. When strength declines, so does your capacity to live independently. Tasks that were once effortless become difficult. You start avoiding activities because they are too hard. Your world shrinks. Your independence erodes.

This is not inevitable. It is preventable. And the tool that prevents it is resistance training.

Resistance training builds muscle mass, and as we discussed in the previous chapter, muscle is the organ of longevity. It regulates blood sugar, supports bone density, produces beneficial signaling molecules, and maintains your resting metabolic rate. But beyond the metabolic benefits, muscle gives you the physical capacity to do things. It is the engine that powers your movement.

Strength training also has unique benefits that cardio does not provide. It increases bone density through mechanical loading. When you lift weights, you create stress on your bones, and your bones respond by becoming denser and stronger. This is critically important for preventing osteoporosis and reducing fracture risk as you age.

Resistance training improves connective tissue health. Your tendons and ligaments adapt to training stress by becoming more resilient. This protects your joints and reduces injury risk. It also improves neuromuscular coordination, the ability of your nervous system to recruit muscle fibers efficiently. This is what allows you to move with control, stability, and power.

Perhaps most importantly, strength training is dose-dependent and progressive. You can start at any level and gradually increase the load over time. This means you can continue to adapt, continue to get stronger, and continue to build capacity for decades. There is no ceiling. Even people in their eighties and nineties can make significant strength gains with proper training.

But what does strength training actually look like in the context of longevity?

It is not about lifting the maximum weight possible. It is not about training to failure on every set. It is not about constantly pushing for personal records at the expense of recovery and joint health.

Longevity-focused strength training is built around fundamental movement patterns: pushing, pulling, hinging, squatting, and carrying. These are the movements that show up in daily life and that preserve functional capacity.

Pushing includes movements like push-ups, bench presses, and overhead presses. These build upper body strength and shoulder stability. Pulling includes rows, pull-ups, and lat pulldowns. These balance the pushing movements and build back strength, which is essential for posture and injury prevention.

Hinging includes deadlifts, Romanian deadlifts, and kettlebell swings. These teach you to move from your hips, load your posterior chain, and lift safely. The hip hinge is one of the most important movement patterns for longevity because it protects your lower back and builds the glutes and hamstrings that support your spine.

Squatting includes goblet squats, back squats, front squats, and split squats. These build leg strength, improve mobility, and train the pattern you use every time you sit down and stand up. The ability to squat deeply and rise without assistance is one of the best predictors of functional capacity in older adults.

Carrying includes farmer's walks, suitcase carries, and loaded carries. These build grip strength, core stability, and the ability to move while holding weight. Carrying is one of the most functional forms of strength training because it directly translates to real-world tasks.

These movement patterns should form the foundation of your strength training program. You do not need dozens of exercises. You need a handful of well-executed movements performed consistently over time with progressive loading.

Progressive overload is the key principle. Your body adapts to the stress you place on it, but only if that stress increases over time. If you lift the same weight for the same reps every week, your body has no reason to adapt. You maintain, but you do not improve.

Progressive overload does not mean adding weight every single session. It means gradually increasing the training stimulus over weeks and months. This can be done by adding weight, increasing reps, adding sets, slowing the tempo, or improving technique. The goal is consistent, sustainable progress, not reckless acceleration.

Equally important is training with good technique. Poor form not only limits your progress but also increases injury risk. Learning to move well, with control and full range of motion, is more important than lifting heavy weight with compensatory patterns. Quality always trumps quantity.

Strength training also needs to be balanced with adequate recovery. Your muscles do not grow during the workout. They grow during the recovery period afterward, when your body repairs the damage and rebuilds tissue stronger than before. Training too frequently without rest leads to overtraining, stagnation, and injury.

For most people, two to four strength training sessions per week is optimal. This provides enough stimulus to drive adaptation while allowing sufficient recovery between sessions. Each session should last forty-five to seventy-five minutes and should target different movement patterns or muscle groups to allow recovery while maintaining frequency.

Strength is the foundation of everything else in longevity training. It preserves muscle, supports metabolic health, protects bones and joints, and maintains the physical capacity to live independently. It is not optional. It is the first priority.

If you do nothing else, lift weights. Do it consistently, progressively, and with good technique. Your future self will thank you.

Zone 2 Cardio Explained Simply

Cardiovascular training is often misunderstood. Most people think of cardio as something you do to burn calories or lose weight. They associate it with long, boring treadmill sessions or brutal high-intensity intervals that leave them gasping for air.

But cardiovascular training, done correctly, is one of the most powerful tools for metabolic health, mitochondrial function, and longevity. The key is understanding what type of cardio to do, how much to do, and why.

Let's start with Zone 2.

Zone 2 refers to a specific intensity of aerobic exercise, typically measured by heart rate or perceived effort. It is the intensity at which you can sustain a conversation but not sing comfortably. You are working, but you are not breathless. You can maintain this pace for extended periods, often an hour or more.

In physiological terms, Zone 2 is the intensity at which your body primarily uses fat for fuel and produces energy aerobically, meaning with oxygen. At this intensity, your mitochondria, the energy-producing structures in your cells, are working efficiently. You are not producing excessive lactate, the byproduct of anaerobic metabolism that causes that burning sensation in your muscles during high-intensity work.

Why does Zone 2 matter for longevity?

First, it improves mitochondrial health. Mitochondria are often called the powerhouses of the cell because they produce the ATP that fuels every cellular process in your body. As you age, mitochondrial function declines. Your mitochondria become less efficient, produce less energy, and generate more oxidative stress. This decline contributes to fatigue, metabolic dysfunction, and aging itself.

Zone 2 training stimulates mitochondrial biogenesis, the creation of new mitochondria. It also improves the efficiency of existing mitochondria. Over time, this makes your cells better at producing energy, which translates to better endurance, faster recovery, and improved metabolic health.

Second, Zone 2 training improves fat oxidation. When you train in Zone 2, your body learns to use fat as fuel more efficiently. This is beneficial not just for body composition, but for metabolic health. The ability to oxidize fat is a marker of metabolic flexibility, the capacity to switch between burning carbohydrates and burning fat depending on availability and demand.

People with poor metabolic flexibility, often those with insulin resistance, are stuck burning primarily carbohydrates. They cannot access their fat stores efficiently. They experience energy crashes when blood sugar drops. They struggle with hunger and cravings. Zone 2 training improves metabolic flexibility, making you more resilient and less dependent on constant carbohydrate intake.

Third, Zone 2 training improves insulin sensitivity. Aerobic exercise, particularly sustained moderate-intensity work, enhances your muscles' ability to take up glucose. This is one of the most effective interventions for preventing and reversing insulin resistance.

Fourth, Zone 2 training is sustainable. Unlike high-intensity interval training, which is demanding and requires significant recovery, Zone 2 is low-stress. You can do it frequently without exceeding your recovery capacity. It supports your strength training rather than interfering with it. It is the foundation of your aerobic base, the cardiovascular fitness that allows you to sustain effort over time.

How much Zone 2 should you do?

For most people, three to four hours per week of Zone 2 training is a reasonable target. This can be broken into three to five sessions of forty-five to sixty minutes each. The specific modality does not matter as much as consistency. Walking, cycling, rowing, swimming, or using an elliptical all work, as long as you maintain the appropriate intensity.

The key is to stay in Zone 2. This requires discipline because Zone 2 feels easy, almost too easy. Most people, when they start cardio, push too hard. They drift into Zone 3 or Zone 4, where the effort feels more substantial and they feel like they are working harder. But this defeats the purpose. Zone 2 is about building aerobic capacity without accumulating fatigue. It is about training your mitochondria, not your willpower.

How do you know if you are in Zone 2? The most accurate method is to use a heart rate monitor and stay within the appropriate heart rate range, which is typically sixty to seventy percent of your maximum heart rate. But you do not need technology. The talk test works just as well. If you can hold a conversation without gasping for air, you are likely in Zone 2. If you cannot talk in full sentences, you are working too hard.

Zone 2 is not glamorous. It is not intense. It will not leave you drenched in sweat or gasping on the floor. But it works. It builds the aerobic base that supports everything else you do. It improves metabolic health in ways that few other interventions can match. And it is sustainable for decades.

This is the foundation of your cardiovascular training. Build it patiently, consistently, and without rushing. The benefits compound over time.

VO₂ Max Relevance (Without Testing Obsession)

If strength is the currency of longevity, VO₂ max is the bank account.

VO₂ max is the maximum amount of oxygen your body can use during exercise. It is measured in milliliters of oxygen per kilogram of body weight per minute. It reflects the combined capacity of your heart, lungs, blood vessels, and muscles to deliver and use oxygen.

Why does this matter? Because VO₂ max is one of the strongest predictors of all-cause mortality. Higher VO₂ max is associated with lower risk of cardiovascular disease, metabolic disease, and early death. The relationship is dose-dependent, meaning the higher your VO₂ max, the lower your risk. Even modest improvements in VO₂ max produce significant reductions in mortality risk.

Studies show that moving from the bottom twenty percent of VO₂ max for your age and sex to the top twenty percent can reduce your risk of death by more than fifty percent. Few interventions, pharmaceutical or otherwise, can match that effect size.

VO₂ max also reflects your functional capacity. It determines how much physical work you can do before fatigue sets in. Higher VO₂ max means you can hike longer, climb stairs without getting winded, play with your grandchildren without exhaustion, and recover quickly from exertion.

As you age, VO₂ max declines unless you maintain it. The average person loses about ten percent per decade after age thirty. This decline is not benign. It is directly associated with reduced quality of life, loss of independence, and increased mortality.

But the decline is not inevitable. VO₂ max is highly trainable at any age. With consistent aerobic training, particularly training that includes higher-intensity work, you can maintain or even improve your VO₂ max well into older age.

Here is the important point: you do not need to formally test your VO₂ max to benefit from training it. Formal VO₂ max testing requires specialized equipment and is typically done in a lab or clinical setting. It is useful for athletes or people who want precise data, but it is not necessary for most people.

What matters is that you include training that challenges your cardiovascular system at higher intensities. This means going beyond Zone 2 and incorporating interval work that pushes you into Zone 4 or Zone 5, where you are breathing hard, your heart rate is elevated, and you cannot sustain the effort for long.

High-intensity interval training, often called HIIT, is the most effective way to improve VO₂ max. A typical HIIT session involves repeated bouts of hard effort, lasting anywhere from thirty seconds to five minutes, followed by recovery periods of equal or longer duration. The hard intervals should feel challenging. You should not be able to hold a conversation. But they should not be all-out sprints that leave you unable to complete the workout.

One or two high-intensity sessions per week, combined with your regular Zone 2 training, is sufficient for most people to maintain or improve VO₂ max. These sessions should be relatively short, typically twenty to thirty minutes including warm-up and cool-down, and should be done on days when you are well-rested and recovered.

The modality matters less than the effort. You can do intervals on a bike, rower, treadmill, or even by running hills. Choose something that allows you to push hard without excessive impact or injury risk. Cycling and rowing are particularly good choices for people with joint issues.

It is important to approach high-intensity work with caution, especially if you are new to training or returning after a long break. High-intensity intervals are demanding. They create significant cardiovascular and metabolic stress. They require adequate recovery. Jumping into hard interval work without a solid aerobic base is a recipe for injury, overtraining, or burnout.

Build your Zone 2 base first. Spend at least several weeks, or even months, building aerobic capacity with moderate-intensity work. Once you have a foundation, add intervals gradually. Start with shorter, less intense intervals and progress over time. Listen to your body. If you are excessively fatigued, not recovering between sessions, or experiencing declining performance, you are doing too much.

VO_2 max is a powerful marker of longevity, but it is not the only one. You do not need to obsess over it. You do not need to test it regularly. You just need to include enough high-intensity work to maintain your cardiovascular capacity. Combined with Zone 2 training, this creates a balanced approach to cardiovascular fitness that will serve you for decades.

Your heart, like your muscles, adapts to the demands you place on it. If you demand nothing, it weakens. If you demand endurance, it builds endurance. If you demand power, it builds power. Train it well, and it will carry you far.

Mobility and Joint Integrity

Strength and cardiovascular fitness get most of the attention in fitness discussions, but mobility and joint integrity are just as important for longevity. Without them, you cannot move well. And if you cannot move well, you cannot train consistently. And if you cannot train consistently, everything else falls apart.

Mobility is the ability to move your joints through their full range of motion with control. It is not the same as flexibility, which is passive range of motion. Mobility is active. It requires not just the ability to reach a position, but the strength and control to move into and out of that position safely.

Good mobility allows you to squat deeply, reach overhead without compensating, rotate your spine without pain, and move fluidly through space. It is the foundation of efficient movement. When you have good mobility, you can train with full range of motion, which maximizes the effectiveness of your strength training and reduces injury risk.

Poor mobility, on the other hand, forces your body to compensate. If your hips are tight, your lower back compensates during squats. If your shoulders are immobile, your neck and upper back compensate during overhead movements. These compensations create inefficient movement patterns, increase stress on joints, and lead to pain and injury over time.

Mobility declines with age if you do nothing to maintain it. Connective tissue becomes stiffer. Joint capsules tighten. Movement patterns become restricted. This is not inevitable, but it is common, especially in sedentary populations.

The good news is that mobility is trainable. With consistent practice, you can maintain or even improve your range of motion well into older age. The key is to include mobility work as a regular part of your training routine, not as an occasional afterthought.

Mobility work does not need to be complicated. It can be as simple as spending five to ten minutes before or after your strength training moving through dynamic stretches, joint circles, and controlled articular rotations. The goal is to move your joints through their full range of motion in a controlled, intentional way.

Examples include hip circles, leg swings, arm circles, spinal rotations, deep squats, and lunges with reaches. These movements prepare your body for training, improve joint health, and reinforce good movement patterns. They do not need to be intense or painful. They just need to be consistent.

Joint integrity is closely related to mobility but focuses specifically on the health and stability of the joint structures themselves. Your joints are complex systems of bones, cartilage, ligaments, tendons, and synovial fluid. They are designed to move, but they are also designed to be stable. The balance between mobility and stability determines joint health.

Resistance training, when done with good technique and appropriate loads, improves joint integrity. It strengthens the muscles that support and stabilize your joints. It increases the resilience of your tendons and ligaments. It stimulates cartilage health through controlled loading.

But resistance training can also damage joints if done poorly. Lifting with poor technique, using excessive loads, or training through pain all increase the risk of joint injury. This is why learning to move well is so important. Technique is not just about maximizing performance. It is about protecting your body so you can train for decades.

Certain joints require extra attention as you age. The shoulders, knees, and lower back are particularly vulnerable to injury and degeneration. Including exercises that specifically strengthen and stabilize these areas is essential for long-term joint health.

For the shoulders, this means including rotator cuff work, scapular stabilization exercises, and movements that build balanced strength in all directions. For the knees, this means strengthening the quadriceps, hamstrings, and glutes, as well as including single-leg work to improve stability. For the lower back, this means building core strength, hip mobility, and proper hinge mechanics.

Mobility and joint integrity are not glamorous. They do not produce visible results in the mirror. They do not give you the same satisfaction as adding weight to the bar. But they are the foundation that allows everything else to work. Without them, your training becomes unsustainable. With them, you can train for life.

Think of mobility and joint integrity as preventative maintenance. You do not wait for your car to break down before you change the oil. You do not wait for your joints to hurt before you address mobility. You build these practices into your routine from the beginning, and you maintain them consistently over time.

Your joints are non-renewable resources. Once damaged, they are difficult or impossible to fully repair. The time to protect them is now, while they are still healthy. Move well, move often, and move with intention. Your joints will reward you with decades of pain-free movement.

Why Rest Is Part of Training

One of the biggest mistakes people make in fitness is thinking that more is always better. They train hard every day, push through fatigue, ignore signs of overtraining, and wonder why they are not progressing. They confuse effort with effectiveness. They mistake exhaustion for accomplishment.

But progress does not happen during training. It happens during recovery.

When you train, you create stress. You damage muscle fibers, deplete energy stores, fatigue your nervous system, and trigger an inflammatory response. This is not bad. This is the stimulus for adaptation. But the stimulus alone is not enough. Your body needs time and resources to respond to that stimulus, to repair the damage, and to rebuild stronger than before.

This is the principle of supercompensation. You stress your body with training. You recover. During recovery, your body adapts by becoming stronger, more resilient, and more capable than it was before. Then you train again, applying a slightly greater stress, and the cycle repeats.

If you skip the recovery phase and train again before your body has adapted, you do not get stronger. You get weaker. You accumulate fatigue. You increase injury risk. You disrupt the hormonal and immune systems that support adaptation. Over time, this leads to overtraining syndrome, a state of chronic fatigue, declining performance, and increased susceptibility to illness.

Rest is not the absence of training. It is an active part of the training process. It is when your body rebuilds. It is when your nervous system resets. It is when your immune system clears debris and repairs tissue. It is when your hormones rebalance.

There are two types of rest: passive and active. Passive rest is complete rest, days when you do nothing physically demanding. These are essential, especially after hard training sessions. Your body needs time to recover fully without additional stress.

Active rest is light movement that promotes recovery without adding significant stress. This includes easy walking, gentle stretching, yoga, swimming, or any low-intensity activity that increases blood flow and helps clear metabolic waste without fatiguing you. Active rest days keep you moving while allowing recovery to continue.

Most people need at least one or two full rest days per week, and possibly more if they are training hard or dealing with life stress. Rest days are not a sign of weakness. They are a sign of intelligence. They are the difference between sustainable progress and eventual breakdown.

Sleep is the most important form of recovery, and we will cover it in detail in a later chapter. For now, understand that sleep is when most of your body's repair and adaptation processes occur. Without adequate sleep, recovery is incomplete. You cannot out-train poor sleep. You cannot supplement your way around it. Sleep is non-negotiable.

Nutrition also plays a critical role in recovery. Your body needs adequate protein to repair muscle tissue, sufficient carbohydrates to replenish glycogen, and healthy fats to support hormone production and reduce inflammation. Eating to support recovery is just as important as eating to fuel training.

Stress management matters too. Psychological stress triggers the same physiological stress response as physical training. If your life is chronically stressful, your body is in a constant state of arousal. Your cortisol is elevated. Your immune system is suppressed. Your recovery is impaired. Managing stress is not a luxury. It is a necessity for long-term progress.

Learning to listen to your body is one of the most important skills you can develop. Your body gives you feedback constantly. Persistent soreness, poor sleep, elevated resting heart rate, declining performance, irritability, frequent illness, and loss of motivation are all signs that your recovery is not keeping pace with your training.

When you notice these signs, the answer is not to push harder. The answer is to rest more. This requires humility and patience. It requires trusting that rest is productive, not wasted time. It requires resisting the cultural pressure to always be doing more.

Training for longevity is not about maximizing short-term performance. It is about sustainable progress over decades. That requires balancing training stress with recovery capacity. It requires building a system that you can maintain not just for months, but for years and decades.

Rest is not optional. It is not something you do when you have time. It is a fundamental part of the training process. Without it, progress stops. With it, everything else works.

Train hard when you train. Rest deeply when you rest. Respect both equally. This is how you build a body that lasts.

This chapter has introduced you to the framework for training that supports longevity. You now understand that longevity training is different from performance training. It is not about how hard you can push today, but about how well you can move for the next fifty years.

You have learned that strength is the foundation of longevity. It preserves muscle, supports metabolic health, protects bones and joints, and maintains the physical capacity to live independently. Strength training built around fundamental movement patterns, performed consistently with progressive overload and good technique, is non-negotiable.

You now understand Zone 2 cardio and why it matters. Zone 2 training improves mitochondrial health, fat oxidation, insulin sensitivity, and aerobic capacity. It is sustainable, low-stress, and forms the foundation of your cardiovascular fitness. Three to four hours per week of Zone 2 training is a reasonable target for most people.

You have learned that VO_2 max is one of the strongest predictors of longevity. Higher VO_2 max is associated with lower mortality risk and better functional capacity. You do not need to test it obsessively, but you do need to include high-intensity interval work one or two times per week to maintain or improve it.

You now know that mobility and joint integrity are essential for sustainable training. Good mobility allows you to move well and train effectively. Joint health protects you from injury and allows you to train for decades. Mobility work and joint-friendly training practices should be integrated into your routine from the beginning.

Finally, you have learned that rest is not the opposite of training but an essential part of it. Recovery is when adaptation happens. Without adequate rest, sleep, nutrition, and stress management, training breaks you down rather than building you up. Balancing training stress with recovery capacity is the key to sustainable progress.

Before moving to Part II, take a moment to reflect on your current training. Do you prioritize strength? Do you include enough Zone 2 cardio? Are you doing any high-intensity work? Do you move well? Are you recovering adequately? Where are your gaps?

These questions will help you understand where to focus as you design your longevity fitness plan. Training for the long game is not complicated, but it requires intention, consistency, and respect for the principles that make progress sustainable.

You are not training for next month. You are training for the next fifty years. Keep that perspective, and everything else falls into place.

CHAPTER 4: EATING FOR STABILITY, NOT RESTRICTION

The diet industry has done something remarkable: it has taken one of life's most fundamental, pleasurable, and necessary activities and turned it into a source of anxiety, confusion, and shame.

Everywhere you turn, there is a new rule. Eat this, not that. Cut carbs. No, cut fat. Fast for sixteen hours. No, eat six small meals. Avoid sugar. Count calories. Track macros. Eliminate entire food groups. Follow rigid meal plans. Weigh your food. Measure your body. Judge yourself by the number on the scale.

It is exhausting. And it does not work.

The vast majority of diets fail. Not because people lack willpower or discipline, but because diets are designed to fail. They are built on restriction, deprivation, and short-term thinking. They ignore the biological, psychological, and social realities of eating. They treat food as the enemy and your body as something to be controlled rather than supported.

This chapter is not about dieting. It is about eating in a way that supports stability, energy, and metabolic health without obsession, restriction, or shame. It is about building a sustainable relationship with food that you can maintain for decades, not just weeks.

If you have spent years jumping from one diet to another, this will feel different. It will feel less rigid. Less prescriptive. Less punishing. That is intentional. Longevity is not built on extremes. It is built on practices you can sustain for the rest of your life.

Let's start by understanding why diets fail and what we can do instead.

Why Diets Fail Long-Term

The logic of dieting seems straightforward: if you eat less than you burn, you will lose weight. This is true in the short term. Create a calorie deficit, and the number on the scale goes down. This is the promise that sells millions of diet books, meal plans, and weight loss programs.

But weight loss is not the same as fat loss. And short-term results are not the same as long-term success.

When you restrict calories significantly, your body does not just burn fat. It also burns muscle. The more aggressive the restriction, the more muscle you lose. This is a disaster for metabolic health and longevity. As we have discussed, muscle is the organ of longevity. Losing muscle makes you weaker, slows your metabolism, impairs insulin sensitivity, and increases your risk of chronic disease.

Beyond muscle loss, severe calorie restriction triggers a cascade of metabolic adaptations designed to protect you from starvation. Your metabolic rate slows. Your hunger hormones, particularly ghrelin, increase. Your satiety hormones, particularly leptin, decrease. Your body becomes more efficient at storing fat and less efficient at burning it.

These adaptations are not a sign that your body is broken. They are a sign that it is working exactly as designed. For most of human history, food scarcity was a real threat. Your body evolved to defend against weight loss by slowing metabolism and increasing hunger. This is a survival mechanism, and it is extremely powerful.

The result is that as soon as you stop restricting, which you inevitably will because restriction is not sustainable, your body is primed to regain weight. You are hungrier than before. Your metabolism is slower than before. Your body is more efficient at storing fat. The weight comes back, often with interest. This is not a failure of willpower. It is biology.

This cycle of restriction and regain, often called yo-yo dieting, is not benign. Each cycle makes the next one harder. You lose muscle with each restriction phase and regain primarily fat. Over time, your body composition worsens, your metabolism slows further, and your relationship with food becomes increasingly dysfunctional.

Then there is the psychological toll. Diets frame food as good or bad, you as disciplined or weak, and your body as something to be controlled. They create a constant state of vigilance, where every meal is a test and every deviation is a failure. This is not a way to live. It is a recipe for disordered eating, anxiety, and shame.

Diets also ignore the social and emotional dimensions of eating. Food is not just fuel. It is culture, connection, comfort, and celebration. Rigid meal plans and food restrictions disconnect you from these aspects of eating, making food a source of stress rather than joy.

The fundamental problem with diets is that they are temporary interventions designed to produce short-term results. They are not systems you can live with. They are not practices that support long-term health. They are Band-Aids on a problem that requires a different approach entirely.

So what is the alternative?

The alternative is eating for stability rather than restriction. It is building a sustainable way of eating that supports your metabolism, preserves muscle, provides consistent energy, and allows you to enjoy food without guilt or obsession. It is about working with your body, not against it.

This approach does not promise rapid weight loss. It does not promise transformation in thirty days. What it promises is something far more valuable: a way of eating you can maintain for the rest of your life, one that supports health, capacity, and longevity rather than undermining them.

Energy Balance Without Counting Forever

Energy balance is real. If you consistently consume more energy than you expend, you will gain weight. If you consistently consume less energy than you expend, you will lose weight. This is thermodynamics, and it cannot be ignored.

But energy balance is not as simple as calories in, calories out. The quality of the calories matters. The macronutrient composition matters. The timing matters. Your activity level matters. Your sleep matters. Your stress levels matter. Your metabolic health matters. All of these factors influence how your body processes and uses the food you eat.

Moreover, precise calorie counting is neither necessary nor sustainable for most people. It is tedious, time-consuming, and often inaccurate. Food labels can be off by up to twenty percent. Portion sizes vary. Your actual energy expenditure fluctuates based on activity, sleep, stress, and metabolic state. Trying to track everything precisely creates an illusion of control that does not actually exist.

The goal is not to count calories forever. The goal is to develop awareness of portion sizes, energy density, and hunger cues so that you can regulate your intake naturally without obsessive tracking.

This starts with understanding energy density. Some foods contain a lot of calories in a small volume. These are energy-dense foods. Examples include oils, butter, nuts, seeds, cheese, and most processed foods. Other foods contain relatively few calories in a large volume. These are low energy-density foods. Examples include vegetables, fruits, lean proteins, and legumes.

Energy-dense foods are not bad. They are nutrient-dense, satisfying, and play an important role in a healthy diet. But they are easy to overeat because they do not fill you up relative to their calorie content. A handful of nuts can contain two hundred calories and barely register in your stomach. A large salad with lean protein can contain the same calories and leave you completely satisfied.

The key is balance. Build meals around low energy-density foods like vegetables and lean proteins, which provide volume, fiber, and satiety. Add smaller amounts of energy-dense foods like oils, nuts, and cheese for flavor, satisfaction, and nutrient diversity. This allows you to eat satisfying portions without consuming excessive calories.

Portion awareness is the next piece. You do not need to weigh and measure everything, but you do need a general sense of what appropriate portions look like. A serving of protein is roughly the size of your palm. A serving of carbohydrates is roughly the size of your cupped hand. A serving of fat is roughly the size of your thumb.

These are not precise measurements. They are visual guides that allow you to build balanced meals without obsessive tracking. Over time, this becomes intuitive. You learn what a balanced plate looks like. You learn how much food leaves you satisfied without being overfull. You learn to adjust based on activity level and hunger.

Hunger itself is a powerful signal, but only if you learn to distinguish between true physical hunger and other types of eating. We will explore this more in the next section, but for now, understand that not all urges to eat are the same. Physical hunger is a signal that your body needs fuel. Other types of eating, driven by boredom, stress, habit, or emotion, are not about fuel at all.

Learning to eat in response to physical hunger, and to stop when satisfied rather than stuffed, is one of the most powerful skills you can develop. It requires slowing down, paying attention, and trusting your body's signals rather than following external rules.

Energy balance, approached this way, is not about rigid restriction. It is about awareness, balance, and flexibility. Some days you will eat more. Some days you will eat less. Over time, if you are eating mostly whole foods, prioritizing protein, managing portions, and responding to hunger cues, your intake will naturally align with your needs.

This is not a quick fix. It is a long-term practice. It requires patience, self-compassion, and a willingness to learn. But it is the only approach that works sustainably. You cannot count calories forever. You can build awareness that lasts a lifetime.

Hunger vs Appetite

Hunger and appetite are not the same thing, although we use the words interchangeably. Understanding the difference is essential for developing a healthy relationship with food.

Hunger is a physiological signal. It is your body's way of telling you that it needs fuel. True hunger builds gradually. It is accompanied by physical sensations: an empty feeling in your stomach, low energy, difficulty concentrating, sometimes irritability. It is satisfied by eating, and it goes away once you have consumed enough food.

Appetite, on the other hand, is a psychological desire to eat. It is not about physical need. It is about wanting food for reasons other than fuel. You can have appetite even when you are not hungry. You can have appetite immediately after eating a full meal.

Appetite is triggered by external cues: the sight or smell of food, the time of day, social situations, stress, boredom, or emotions. It is also influenced by food palatability. Highly palatable foods, those that are engineered to be hyper-rewarding with combinations of fat, sugar, and salt, activate the reward centers in your brain and drive eating beyond physical need.

The modern food environment is designed to stimulate appetite. Food is everywhere, highly palatable, aggressively marketed, and available twenty-four hours a day. This creates a constant state of food availability and food cues that our brains are not equipped to handle. We are surrounded by appetite triggers, and most of us have lost touch with true physical hunger.

Learning to distinguish between hunger and appetite is a skill that requires practice. It starts with asking a simple question before you eat: am I physically hungry, or am I eating for another reason?

If you are physically hungry, eat. Choose foods that will satisfy you and provide sustained energy. If you are not physically hungry, pause and investigate. What is driving the desire to eat? Are you bored? Stressed? Tired? Lonely? Seeking comfort or distraction?

This is not about judging yourself. It is about awareness. Once you understand what is driving the urge to eat, you can address the actual need. If you are stressed, food will not fix the stress. It might provide temporary comfort, but it will not solve the underlying problem. If you are tired, food will not give you energy. You need rest, not calories.

Sometimes you will choose to eat even when you are not physically hungry, and that is okay. Food is more than fuel. It is pleasure, connection, and culture. Eating for enjoyment, in social settings, or as part of celebrations is a normal and healthy part of life. The key is doing so consciously, without guilt, and without it becoming your default response to every uncomfortable emotion.

The problem arises when eating becomes the primary strategy for managing emotions, stress, or discomfort. This is called emotional eating, and we will address it in the next section. For now, understand that eating in response to appetite rather than hunger is not inherently bad. It becomes problematic only when it is unconscious, habitual, and disconnected from your actual needs.

One of the most effective ways to reconnect with physical hunger is to create regular meal spacing. Instead of grazing throughout the day, eat structured meals with at least three to four hours between them. This allows your blood sugar and insulin to return to baseline. It allows your stomach to empty. It allows true physical hunger to emerge.

When you eat your next meal, pay attention to how it feels. Are you genuinely hungry, or are you eating out of habit or schedule? How much food does it take to satisfy your hunger? What does satisfaction feel like, as opposed to being stuffed?

These questions help you develop hunger awareness, the ability to recognize and respond to your body's actual fuel needs. Over time, this becomes intuitive. You learn to trust your hunger. You learn that it is okay to feel hungry before meals. You learn that hunger is not an emergency that needs to be fixed immediately with the nearest available food.

Rebuilding this connection takes time, especially if you have spent years ignoring hunger signals, eating on external schedules, or restricting food to the point where hunger becomes distorted. Be patient with yourself. This is not a skill you develop overnight. It is a practice that deepens over time.

Hunger is information. It is not something to fear or suppress. It is a signal that your body is working as designed. Learning to listen to it, trust it, and respond to it appropriately is one of the foundations of sustainable eating.

Satiety Signals

If hunger tells you when to start eating, satiety tells you when to stop. But like hunger, satiety is a signal that most people have learned to ignore.

Satiety is the feeling of fullness and satisfaction that follows eating. It is not just about your stomach being physically full. It is a complex signal involving your stomach, intestines, hormones, and brain. When functioning properly, satiety allows you to stop eating when you have had enough, even if food is still available.

But satiety takes time. It takes approximately fifteen to twenty minutes for the signal to travel from your stomach to your brain. If you eat quickly, you can consume far more food than you need before the satiety signal registers. This is one reason why eating slowly is such a powerful practice.

Satiety is also influenced by the macronutrient composition of your meal. Protein is the most satiating macronutrient, followed by fiber, fat, and carbohydrates. This is why meals built around protein and vegetables keep you satisfied longer than meals built around refined carbohydrates.

High-protein meals trigger the release of satiety hormones like peptide YY and glucagon-like peptide-1, which signal fullness to your brain. They also suppress ghrelin, the hunger hormone. This is one reason why increasing protein intake is such an effective strategy for managing appetite and body composition without conscious restriction.

Fiber also plays a critical role in satiety. Fiber adds bulk to your meals without adding many calories. It slows digestion, which prolongs the feeling of fullness. It stabilizes blood sugar, preventing the crashes that trigger hunger. Meals rich in vegetables, fruits, whole grains, and legumes are naturally more satiating than meals low in fiber.

Fat contributes to satiety as well, although the effect is less immediate than protein. Fat slows gastric emptying, meaning it keeps food in your stomach longer. This prolongs the feeling of fullness between meals. However, because fat is energy-dense, it is easy to overconsume. This is why balancing fat with protein and fiber is important.

Beyond macronutrients, the act of eating itself influences satiety. Eating slowly, chewing thoroughly, and paying attention to your food all enhance satiety. When you eat mindfully, you give your body time to register fullness. You notice subtle signals that tell you when you have had enough. You stop eating at satisfaction rather than discomfort.

In contrast, eating quickly, while distracted, or while multitasking disconnects you from satiety signals. You eat past fullness without noticing. You finish your plate out of habit rather than need. You continue eating because the food is in front of you, not because you are still hungry.

Learning to eat to satisfaction, not to fullness, is one of the most important skills for long-term weight management and metabolic health. Satisfaction is the point at which you feel pleasantly full, energized, and content. You could eat more, but you do not need to. Fullness, or worse, being stuffed, is uncomfortable. It is the feeling of having eaten too much.

The difference is subtle but significant. Stopping at satisfaction means you have eaten enough to meet your needs without exceeding them. Stopping at fullness means you have eaten past your needs. Over time, consistently eating to fullness rather than satisfaction leads to weight gain and metabolic dysfunction.

How do you learn to recognize satiety and stop at satisfaction? The answer is practice and attention.

Start by eating without distractions. Put away your phone. Turn off the TV. Sit down at a table. Focus on your food. Notice the flavors, textures, and aromas. Chew thoroughly. Eat slowly.

Halfway through your meal, pause. Check in with yourself. How hungry are you now? Are you still physically hungry, or are you eating out of habit? Could you stop here and feel satisfied?

This pause is not about restriction. It is about awareness. Sometimes you will realize you are still hungry and continue eating. Other times you will realize you are satisfied and choose to stop. Both are fine. The goal is to make the decision consciously rather than automatically.

Over time, this practice becomes automatic. You develop an internal sense of when you have had enough. You trust your body to tell you when to stop. You no longer need external rules or portion control because you are regulating intake naturally based on satiety signals.

This is one of the most liberating aspects of eating for stability rather than restriction. You do not need to finish your plate. You do not need to eat a predetermined portion. You eat until you are satisfied, and you stop. The food will still be there later if you get hungry again.

Satiety is not the enemy. It is a tool. It is your body's way of helping you regulate intake without conscious effort. Learning to listen to it, trust it, and respond to it is essential for building a sustainable relationship with food.

Emotional Eating Without Shame

Let's be honest: everyone eats emotionally sometimes. Food is comforting. It is familiar. It is soothing. When you are stressed, tired, lonely, or anxious, food offers a quick, reliable source of relief. There is nothing inherently wrong with this.

The problem arises when emotional eating becomes your primary coping mechanism, when it is frequent, unconscious, and disconnected from physical hunger. When every difficult emotion triggers eating, food stops being a source of nourishment and becomes a way to avoid feeling.

Emotional eating is not a character flaw. It is not a sign of weakness or lack of discipline. It is a learned behavior, often developed in childhood, that served a purpose at some point. Food was available when other forms of comfort were not. It was reliable when people were not. It was safe when the world was not.

Understanding this is the first step toward changing the pattern. You are not broken. You are not failing. You are using a tool that worked in the past but may not be serving you well in the present.

The goal is not to eliminate emotional eating entirely. The goal is to develop awareness around it, reduce its frequency, and expand your repertoire of coping strategies so that food is not the only tool you have.

Start by noticing when emotional eating happens. What triggers it? Stress at work? Conflict in relationships? Boredom at night? Loneliness? Fatigue? Anxiety about the future?

Keep a simple journal for a week or two. When you find yourself eating outside of physical hunger, pause and write down what you were feeling just before the urge to eat. Do not judge it. Just notice it. Patterns will emerge.

Once you see the patterns, you can start to address the underlying emotions directly. If stress triggers eating, what else could you do when you feel stressed? Take a walk? Call a friend? Practice breathwork? Write in a journal? These are not distractions. They are alternative coping strategies that address the actual need rather than suppressing it temporarily with food.

This does not mean these strategies will feel as immediately satisfying as eating. They will not, at least not at first. Food provides instant relief. Other coping strategies take time to develop and feel effective. But over time, as you practice them, they become just as reliable, and they do not come with the guilt, discomfort, or metabolic consequences that often follow emotional eating.

It is also important to address the shame around emotional eating. Shame does not help. It makes the problem worse. When you feel ashamed after eating, you are more likely to restrict, which leads to more hunger, which leads to more emotional eating. This is the restrict-binge cycle, and it is driven by shame and judgment.

Instead of shame, practice curiosity and compassion. When you notice yourself eating emotionally, instead of berating yourself, ask: what was I feeling? What did I need in that moment? Did the food help? Is there something else that might have helped more?

This reframe shifts emotional eating from a moral failure to a learning opportunity. Over time, you develop a deeper understanding of your triggers, your needs, and your patterns. This awareness is what allows you to change.

Another important piece is ensuring that you are not physically under-fueled. One of the most common triggers for emotional eating is restriction. When you are chronically underfed, your body is in a state of physiological stress. Your hunger hormones are elevated. Your willpower is depleted. Every emotion feels more intense, and food becomes irresistible.

This is why eating for stability, with adequate protein, regular meals, and sufficient energy, is so important. When you are well-nourished, emotional eating becomes less frequent and less intense. You have the physical and mental resources to cope with emotions in other ways.

Finally, recognize that some emotional eating is normal and acceptable. Food is part of how we celebrate, connect, and comfort ourselves. Eating ice cream after a hard day, baking cookies when you are sad, or sharing a meal with loved ones during difficult times are all healthy expressions of food's role in our lives.

The key is whether eating is your only strategy or one of many. If food is the only tool you have, it becomes a problem. If it is one tool among many, used consciously and without guilt, it is simply part of being human.

Emotional eating without shame means acknowledging it when it happens, understanding why it happened, and choosing to respond with compassion rather than judgment. It means building other coping strategies so you have options. It means ensuring you are physically well-nourished so you are not fighting biology. And it means accepting that food is more than fuel, and that eating for comfort sometimes is part of a full, human life.

This is not a problem to be fixed. It is a pattern to be understood and gently shifted over time.

This chapter has laid the foundation for eating in a way that supports longevity without restriction, obsession, or shame. You now understand why diets fail: they are built on short-term thinking, they cause muscle loss, they trigger metabolic adaptations that make weight regain inevitable, and they damage your relationship with food.

You have learned that energy balance is real, but precise calorie counting is not sustainable. Instead, focus on building awareness of portion sizes, energy density, and hunger cues. Eat mostly whole foods, prioritize protein, manage portions using visual guides, and learn to respond to physical hunger rather than external rules.

You now understand the difference between hunger and appetite. Hunger is a physiological signal that your body needs fuel. Appetite is a psychological desire to eat, triggered by external cues, emotions, or food palatability. Learning to distinguish between them is essential for eating in response to your body's actual needs.

You have learned that satiety is the signal that tells you when to stop eating. It takes time to register, which is why eating slowly and mindfully is so important. Protein, fiber, and fat all contribute to satiety. Learning to stop at satisfaction rather than fullness is one of the most powerful skills for long-term weight management.

Finally, you have learned that emotional eating is not a character flaw. It is a learned behavior that can be understood and gently shifted. The goal is not to eliminate it, but to develop awareness around it, reduce its frequency, and build alternative coping strategies. Approaching emotional eating with curiosity and compassion, rather than shame, is what allows change to happen.

Before moving to Chapter 5, take a moment to reflect on your current eating patterns. Do you eat in response to physical hunger, or are you driven by appetite, emotions, or external cues? Do you eat slowly and stop at satisfaction, or do you eat quickly and finish your plate regardless of hunger? Do you approach eating with awareness and compassion, or with judgment and shame?

These questions are not meant to criticize. They are meant to create awareness. Awareness is the first step toward change. As you continue through this section, you will build on this foundation with specific nutritional principles and practical strategies that support metabolic health and longevity.

Eating for stability is not about perfection. It is about progress. It is about building practices you can sustain for the rest of your life, practices that support your body rather than fighting against it.

CHAPTER 5: LONGEVITY NUTRITION PRINCIPLES

Now that we have established the foundational mindset for eating, it is time to get specific. What should you actually eat to support longevity, preserve muscle, maintain metabolic health, and sustain energy for decades?

This chapter will give you the principles, not rigid rules. Principles are flexible. They adapt to your life, your preferences, and your circumstances. They guide your decisions without controlling them. They allow you to make informed choices rather than following someone else's meal plan.

The principles we will cover are: protein targets by age group, carbohydrate timing for activity, fats for hormone and brain health, fiber and gut health, and hydration strategy. These are the nutritional levers that matter most for longevity. Master these, and the details take care of themselves.

Let's begin with the foundation: protein.

Protein Targets by Age Group

Protein is the most important macronutrient for longevity, and most people, especially as they age, do not consume enough of it.

As we discussed in Chapter 2, protein provides the amino acids your body needs to build and repair tissue. Every day, your body breaks down and rebuilds proteins in a constant cycle of turnover. To maintain this process, you need a steady supply of dietary protein.

When you are young, your body is efficient at using protein. But as you age, particularly after forty, your body develops anabolic resistance. Your muscles become less responsive to the signal to build and repair. You need more protein to stimulate the same muscle protein synthesis response that required less protein when you were younger.

If you do not increase your protein intake as you age, you lose muscle. This is one of the primary drivers of sarcopenia. The typical Western diet, which is often carbohydrate-heavy and protein-light, simply does not provide enough amino acids to prevent muscle loss in older adults.

So how much protein do you need?

For adults under forty who are sedentary or lightly active, the current recommended dietary allowance of 0.8 grams per kilogram of body weight per day may be sufficient to prevent deficiency. But it is not sufficient to optimize muscle maintenance, metabolic health, or longevity.

For adults over forty, especially those who are training regularly, the target should be significantly higher. A reasonable range is 1.6 to 2.2 grams of protein per kilogram of body weight per day, or approximately 0.7 to 1.0 grams per pound of body weight.

Let's break this down by age group and activity level:

Ages 30-50, Sedentary or Lightly Active: Aim for 1.2 to 1.6 grams per kilogram of body weight per day. For a 70-kilogram (154-pound) person, this is approximately 84 to 112 grams of protein per day. This is enough to prevent muscle loss and support basic metabolic functions.

Ages 30-50, Training Regularly: Aim for 1.6 to 2.0 grams per kilogram of body weight per day. For a 70-kilogram person, this is approximately 112 to 140 grams of protein per day. This supports muscle maintenance, recovery from training, and metabolic health.

Ages 50-70, Sedentary or Lightly Active: Aim for 1.4 to 1.8 grams per kilogram of body weight per day. For a 70-kilogram person, this is approximately 98 to 126 grams of protein per day. Anabolic resistance increases in this age range, so higher protein intake is necessary even without regular training.

Ages 50-70, Training Regularly: Aim for 1.8 to 2.2 grams per kilogram of body weight per day. For a 70-kilogram person, this is approximately 126 to 154 grams of protein per day. This higher intake overcomes anabolic resistance and supports muscle maintenance and growth.

Ages 70+: Aim for at least 1.6 to 2.0 grams per kilogram of body weight per day, regardless of activity level. For a 70-kilogram person, this is approximately 112 to 140 grams per day. At this age, preventing muscle loss is critical for maintaining independence and quality of life.

These targets may seem high, especially if you are not used to tracking protein. But they are achievable with intentional meal planning.

Each meal should contain a substantial protein source. Breakfast might include eggs, Greek yogurt, cottage cheese, or a protein shake. Lunch might include chicken, fish, turkey, tofu, or legumes. Dinner might include beef, pork, salmon, or tempeh. Snacks can include protein-rich options like jerky, nuts, protein bars, or more Greek yogurt.

Protein distribution matters as much as total intake. Rather than consuming most of your protein at one meal, distribute it across three to four meals throughout the day. Each meal should contain at least 25 to 40 grams of protein to maximally stimulate muscle protein synthesis.

This pattern is more effective for building and maintaining muscle than eating small amounts of protein throughout the day or loading it all into one meal. Your muscles need repeated signals to build throughout the day, not just one large signal.

Leucine content is also important. Leucine is the primary amino acid that triggers muscle protein synthesis. Animal proteins like meat, poultry, fish, eggs, and dairy are rich in leucine. Plant proteins tend to be lower in leucine, which means vegetarians and vegans need to consume more total protein to achieve the same muscle-building effect.

If you follow a plant-based diet, aim for the higher end of the protein ranges. Combine different plant protein sources to ensure you are getting all essential amino acids. Consider supplementing with essential amino acids or plant-based protein powders that are fortified with leucine.

Protein is not just for building muscle. It is highly satiating, which helps regulate appetite and body composition without conscious restriction. It has a high thermic effect, meaning your body burns more calories digesting and processing it compared to carbohydrates or fats. It supports immune function, hormone production, and tissue repair throughout your body.

If you take one action from this chapter, make it this: increase your protein intake. Track it for one week to see where you currently stand. Most people are surprised to find they are consuming far less than they thought. Then adjust your meals to hit your target consistently.

Use a simple tracking app if needed, but only temporarily. The goal is to build awareness, not to track forever. Once you know what 30 grams of protein looks like at a meal, you can eyeball it moving forward.

Protein is the foundation of longevity nutrition. Everything else builds on this.

Carbohydrate Timing for Activity

Carbohydrates have become one of the most controversial topics in nutrition. Some experts tell you to eat more carbs. Others tell you to eliminate them entirely. The truth, as usual, is more nuanced.

Carbohydrates are not inherently good or bad. They are a tool. When used appropriately, they support performance, recovery, and metabolic health. When misused, they contribute to blood sugar instability, insulin resistance, and fat gain.

The key is matching your carbohydrate intake to your activity level and timing them strategically around training.

Let's start with the basics. Carbohydrates are your body's preferred fuel for high-intensity activity. When you do resistance training, intervals, or any intense physical work, your muscles primarily use glucose for energy. This glucose comes from the carbohydrates you eat, which are stored in your muscles and liver as glycogen.

If you train hard and do not consume adequate carbohydrates, your glycogen stores become depleted. Your performance suffers. Your recovery is impaired. Your body may break down muscle tissue to create glucose through a process called gluconeogenesis. This is the opposite of what you want.

On the other hand, if you consume large amounts of carbohydrates while sedentary, your body has no use for them. Your glycogen stores are already full. The excess glucose gets stored as fat. Your blood sugar spikes and crashes. Your insulin levels remain elevated. Over time, this contributes to insulin resistance and metabolic dysfunction.

This is why carbohydrate timing matters. The goal is to consume more carbohydrates on days when you are active and need them, and fewer carbohydrates on days when you are sedentary and do not.

Here is a practical framework:

High-Carbohydrate Days (Training Days): On days when you do resistance training, high-intensity intervals, or prolonged cardiovascular work, your carbohydrate needs are higher. Aim for approximately 3 to 5 grams of carbohydrates per kilogram of body weight, depending on the volume and intensity of your training.

For a 70-kilogram person, this is roughly 210 to 350 grams of carbohydrates. This might sound like a lot, but it is necessary to support performance and recovery. Include carbohydrates at every meal, with the largest portion in the meal following your training session.

Moderate-Carbohydrate Days (Light Activity Days): On days when you do light activity like walking, yoga, or mobility work, your carbohydrate needs are moderate. Aim for approximately 2 to 3 grams of carbohydrates per kilogram of body weight.

For a 70-kilogram person, this is roughly 140 to 210 grams of carbohydrates. Include carbohydrates at most meals, prioritizing them earlier in the day or around your activity.

Lower-Carbohydrate Days (Rest Days): On complete rest days, when your activity level is minimal, your carbohydrate needs are lower. Aim for approximately 1 to 2 grams of carbohydrates per kilogram of body weight.

For a 70-kilogram person, this is roughly 70 to 140 grams of carbohydrates. Focus on non-starchy vegetables, moderate portions of fruit, and minimal grains or starchy carbohydrates. Prioritize protein and healthy fats to maintain satiety.

This approach, sometimes called carbohydrate cycling, allows you to match fuel intake to fuel demand. You eat more when you need more, and less when you need less. This supports performance, recovery, and body composition without requiring constant restriction.

The timing within the day also matters. The best time to consume carbohydrates is around your training sessions, particularly in the meal immediately following training. This is when your muscles are most insulin-sensitive and most receptive to glucose uptake. Eating carbohydrates post-workout replenishes glycogen stores, supports recovery, and produces a smaller blood sugar spike than eating the same carbohydrates while sedentary.

Eating carbohydrates before training can also be beneficial, particularly for longer or higher-intensity sessions. A meal containing carbohydrates one to three hours before training ensures your glycogen stores are topped off and you have readily available fuel.

Carbohydrates later in the day, particularly in the evening, are often demonized in popular diet culture. The claim is that eating carbs at night makes you fat. This is not true. What matters is total intake and activity level, not the time of day. In fact, eating carbohydrates in the evening can support sleep by increasing serotonin and melatonin production.

The quality of carbohydrates matters as much as the quantity and timing. Prioritize minimally processed carbohydrates that are high in fiber and nutrients: vegetables, fruits, whole grains, legumes, and tubers. These foods produce smaller blood sugar responses, provide sustained energy, and support gut health.

Minimize highly processed carbohydrates that are low in fiber and high in sugar: white bread, pastries, sugary cereals, candy, and most packaged snacks. These foods spike blood sugar, drive insulin resistance, and provide little nutritional value.

This is not about perfection. It is about making better choices most of the time. If you eat a piece of cake at a celebration, it is not a problem. If you eat sugary cereal every morning and cookies every night, it becomes a problem.

Carbohydrate timing is a powerful tool for optimizing performance, recovery, and metabolic health. Match your intake to your activity. Time carbohydrates around training. Choose quality sources. This allows you to enjoy carbohydrates without the negative metabolic consequences that come from misusing them.

Fats for Hormone and Brain Health

Fat has been vilified for decades. We were told that eating fat makes you fat, that fat clogs your arteries, and that low-fat diets are the key to health. This advice was not just wrong. It was harmful.

Fat is essential. Your body needs fat for hormone production, brain function, cell membrane integrity, vitamin absorption, and inflammation regulation. Severely restricting fat, as many low-fat diets recommend, disrupts these critical processes.

The key is not to avoid fat, but to understand which fats to prioritize and which to limit.

Let's start with the essentials. Dietary fat comes in several forms: saturated fat, monounsaturated fat, polyunsaturated fat (including omega-3 and omega-6 fatty acids), and trans fat. Each has different effects on your health.

Monounsaturated Fats: These are found in olive oil, avocados, nuts, and seeds. They are universally recognized as healthy. They improve cholesterol profiles, reduce inflammation, and support cardiovascular health. They should form the foundation of your fat intake.

Polyunsaturated Fats (Omega-3): Omega-3 fatty acids, particularly EPA and DHA, are found in fatty fish like salmon, sardines, and mackerel, as well as in smaller amounts in walnuts, flaxseeds, and chia seeds. Omega-3s are anti-inflammatory, support brain health, improve cardiovascular function, and may reduce the risk of neurodegenerative disease. Most people do not consume enough omega-3s. Aim for at least two servings of fatty fish per week, or consider supplementing with a high-quality fish oil.

Polyunsaturated Fats (Omega-6): Omega-6 fatty acids are found in vegetable oils, nuts, and seeds. They are essential, but the modern diet provides far too much omega-6 relative to omega-3. The ideal ratio is thought to be somewhere between 1:1 and 4:1 (omega-6 to omega-3). The typical Western diet is closer to 15:1 or even 20:1. This imbalance promotes inflammation and contributes to chronic disease. Reduce your intake of processed vegetable oils like soybean, corn, and sunflower oil. Use olive oil, avocado oil, or coconut oil instead.

Saturated Fat: This is where things get controversial. Saturated fat is found in animal products like meat, butter, and cheese, as well as in coconut oil. For decades, we were told that saturated fat causes heart disease. Recent research suggests the relationship is more complex. Saturated fat does raise LDL cholesterol in some people, but not all LDL is equally harmful. The type of LDL matters, and saturated fat primarily raises large, fluffy LDL particles, which are less atherogenic than small, dense particles.

That said, excessive saturated fat intake, particularly in the context of a high-carbohydrate, high-calorie diet, can contribute to metabolic dysfunction. A reasonable approach is to include moderate amounts of saturated fat from whole food sources, while prioritizing monounsaturated and omega-3 fats. Aim for saturated fat to comprise less than ten percent of your total calories.

Trans Fats: These are found in partially hydrogenated oils, which are used in many processed and fried foods. Trans fats are unequivocally harmful. They raise LDL cholesterol, lower HDL cholesterol, promote inflammation, and increase the risk of cardiovascular disease. Avoid them completely. Read labels and avoid any product that contains partially hydrogenated oil.

Beyond the type of fat, the total amount matters. Fat is energy-dense, containing nine calories per gram compared to four calories per gram for protein and carbohydrates. This means it is easy to overconsume fat without realizing it. A tablespoon of oil contains about 120 calories. A handful of nuts can contain 200 calories. A few slices of cheese can add several hundred calories to a meal.

This does not mean you should avoid these foods. They are nutritious, satisfying, and important for health. But you need to be mindful of portions. Use oils in cooking, but measure them rather than pouring freely. Enjoy nuts and seeds, but stick to a small handful rather than eating from the bag. Include cheese and butter, but in moderate amounts.

A reasonable target for total fat intake is approximately 25 to 35 percent of your total calories. For someone consuming 2,000 calories per day, this is roughly 55 to 78 grams of fat. For someone consuming 2,500 calories, this is roughly 69 to 97 grams of fat.

Within this total, prioritize omega-3 fats from fatty fish and plant sources. Use olive oil as your primary cooking and salad oil. Include moderate amounts of nuts, seeds, and avocados. Limit processed vegetable oils and trans fats. Include some saturated fat from whole food sources like eggs, meat, and dairy, but do not make it the dominant fat in your diet.

Fat plays a particularly important role in hormone production. Many hormones, including testosterone, estrogen, and cortisol, are synthesized from cholesterol. Severely restricting fat, especially saturated fat, can impair hormone production and lead to low testosterone, irregular menstrual cycles, and poor stress response.

Fat is also critical for brain health. Your brain is approximately sixty percent fat by dry weight. The myelin sheaths that insulate your neurons are made of fat. DHA, an omega-3 fatty acid, is a major structural component of brain tissue. Adequate fat intake, particularly omega-3s, supports cognitive function, mood regulation, and may reduce the risk of neurodegenerative diseases like Alzheimer's.

Fat also supports the absorption of fat-soluble vitamins: A, D, E, and K. Eating vegetables without any fat means you absorb far fewer of these critical nutrients. This is one reason why extremely low-fat diets, despite being rich in vegetables, can lead to nutrient deficiencies.

Finally, fat contributes to satiety. Meals that contain fat are more satisfying and keep you full longer than low-fat meals. This is why eating fat does not inherently make you fat, despite the calorie density. When you eat adequate fat, you naturally eat less overall because you are satisfied.

The key is balance. Include fat at every meal, but do not overdo it. Prioritize quality fats from whole food sources. Avoid trans fats and excessive processed oils. This approach supports hormone health, brain function, and long-term metabolic health without unnecessary restriction.

Fiber and Gut Health

Fiber is one of the most underappreciated components of a longevity-focused diet. It does not provide calories. It does not build muscle. It is not glamorous or exciting. But it is absolutely essential for metabolic health, gut health, and disease prevention.

Fiber is the indigestible part of plant foods. It passes through your digestive system largely intact, but along the way, it does remarkable things. It slows digestion, stabilizes blood sugar, feeds beneficial gut bacteria, promotes satiety, supports regular bowel movements, and reduces the risk of chronic disease.

There are two types of fiber: soluble and insoluble. Both are important.

Soluble Fiber: This type dissolves in water and forms a gel-like substance in your digestive tract. It slows the absorption of glucose, which blunts blood sugar spikes. It binds to cholesterol and helps remove it from your body, which can improve cardiovascular health. It also feeds beneficial gut bacteria, supporting a healthy microbiome.

Soluble fiber is found in oats, beans, lentils, apples, citrus fruits, carrots, and psyllium husk.

Insoluble Fiber: This type does not dissolve in water. It adds bulk to your stool and helps food move through your digestive system more quickly. It prevents constipation and supports regular bowel movements. It also contributes to satiety by adding volume to meals without adding calories.

Insoluble fiber is found in whole grains, nuts, seeds, vegetables (especially leafy greens and cruciferous vegetables), and the skins of fruits and vegetables.

Most plant foods contain both types of fiber, so you do not need to obsess over getting the perfect ratio. Just eat a variety of plant foods, and you will get both.

The current recommendation for fiber intake is 25 grams per day for women and 38 grams per day for men. However, most people consume far less, averaging only about 15 grams per day. This shortfall has significant health consequences.

Low fiber intake is associated with higher rates of cardiovascular disease, type 2 diabetes, colorectal cancer, and all-cause mortality. High fiber intake, on the other hand, is protective. Studies consistently show that people who consume more fiber live longer and have lower rates of chronic disease.

One of fiber's most important roles is supporting gut health. Your gut is home to trillions of bacteria, collectively called the microbiome. These bacteria influence everything from digestion and metabolism to immune function and mood.

Beneficial gut bacteria feed on fiber, particularly soluble fiber. When they digest fiber, they produce short-chain fatty acids like butyrate, which have anti-inflammatory effects and support the health of your intestinal lining. A healthy, diverse microbiome is associated with better metabolic health, stronger immune function, and lower inflammation.

Conversely, a diet low in fiber starves beneficial bacteria and allows harmful bacteria to proliferate. This imbalance, called dysbiosis, is associated with inflammation, insulin resistance, obesity, and a host of other health problems.

Fiber also plays a critical role in blood sugar management. When you eat carbohydrates with fiber, the fiber slows the digestion and absorption of glucose. This produces a smaller, more gradual rise in blood sugar and a correspondingly smaller insulin response. This is why whole grains, legumes, fruits, and vegetables produce much smaller blood sugar spikes than refined carbohydrates like white bread and pastries.

Fiber also promotes satiety. High-fiber foods take longer to chew and digest, which gives your body time to register fullness. They add bulk to your meals without adding many calories. This is why people who eat high-fiber diets tend to have better appetite control and lower body weight than people who eat low-fiber diets.

How do you increase your fiber intake?

Start by prioritizing whole, minimally processed plant foods. Every meal should include vegetables. Snacks should include fruits, nuts, or seeds. Replace refined grains with whole grains. Choose oats, quinoa, brown rice, and whole wheat over white bread, white rice, and sugary cereals.

Include legumes regularly. Beans, lentils, and chickpeas are some of the most fiber-rich foods available. A single cup of cooked lentils contains about 15 grams of fiber, roughly half the daily target. Add them to soups, salads, stews, or eat them as a side dish.

Leave the skins on fruits and vegetables when possible. The skin is where much of the fiber is concentrated. Eat apples with the skin. Leave the peel on potatoes. Eat whole oranges instead of drinking orange juice.

If you are currently eating very little fiber, increase your intake gradually. A sudden jump from 15 grams to 40 grams per day can cause digestive discomfort, gas, and bloating. Add 5 grams every few days and allow your gut to adapt. Drink plenty of water, as fiber needs water to function properly.

Fiber is not optional for longevity. It is foundational. It supports metabolic health, gut health, satiety, and disease prevention. Make it a priority in every meal, and your body will thank you for decades.

Hydration Strategy

Water is so fundamental to life that we often overlook its importance. But hydration status affects everything: physical performance, cognitive function, temperature regulation, nutrient transport, waste removal, and metabolic health.

Dehydration, even mild dehydration, impairs performance, increases perceived effort, reduces endurance, and slows recovery. Chronic low-level dehydration is associated with kidney problems, constipation, and poor cognitive function.

Yet most people do not drink enough water. They wait until they are thirsty, which means they are already dehydrated. They rely on coffee, tea, and other beverages, many of which have diuretic effects. They confuse thirst with hunger and eat when their body is asking for water.

So how much water do you need?

The old recommendation of eight glasses per day is a reasonable starting point, but individual needs vary based on body size, activity level, climate, and overall health. A more personalized approach is to aim for approximately 30 to 40 milliliters of water per kilogram of body weight per day.

For a 70-kilogram person, this is roughly 2.1 to 2.8 liters, or about 9 to 12 cups. On training days, particularly in hot weather or during intense sessions, you may need more.

The simplest way to assess your hydration status is to look at your urine. Pale yellow urine indicates good hydration. Dark yellow or amber urine indicates dehydration. Clear urine suggests you may be drinking more than necessary, although this is rarely a problem.

Another indicator is frequency. You should be urinating every two to four hours during waking hours. If you go much longer, you are likely not drinking enough. If you are urinating every hour, you may be drinking too much.

Hydration needs increase with training. During exercise, you lose water through sweat. The amount varies based on intensity, duration, temperature, and individual sweat rate. For most people, drinking 500 to 750 milliliters per hour of exercise is sufficient. For longer or more intense sessions, you may need more.

Electrolytes also matter, particularly sodium. When you sweat, you lose not just water but also electrolytes, especially sodium. If you drink large amounts of plain water without replacing electrolytes, you can dilute the sodium in your blood to dangerous levels, a condition called hyponatremia.

For most training sessions under an hour, plain water is fine. For sessions longer than an hour, particularly in hot conditions or if you are a heavy sweater, consider adding electrolytes. This can be as simple as adding a pinch of salt to your water bottle or using an electrolyte supplement.

Timing matters too. Drinking water consistently throughout the day is more effective than chugging large amounts all at once. Your body can only absorb a certain amount of water at a time. Drinking a liter in ten minutes means most of it will be excreted rather than absorbed.

Start your day with water. After a night of sleep, your body is mildly dehydrated. Drinking one or two glasses first thing in the morning rehydrates you, supports digestion, and sets the tone for the day.

Drink water before, during, and after training. Aim to start your training session well-hydrated. Drink during the session if it lasts longer than thirty minutes. Rehydrate afterward by drinking approximately 1.5 times the fluid you lost through sweat. If you do not want to weigh yourself before and after, a reasonable rule is to drink until your urine is pale yellow.

Beyond plain water, other beverages contribute to hydration. Tea and coffee, despite their mild diuretic effects, still provide net hydration. Milk, herbal teas, and broths all count. Fruits and vegetables with high water content, like cucumbers, watermelon, and oranges, also contribute.

What does not help: alcohol and sugary beverages. Alcohol is a diuretic and actively dehydrates you. Sugary drinks like soda and juice provide fluids but also spike blood sugar and contribute empty calories. They are not hydrating choices.

Hydration is simple but not trivial. Drink water consistently throughout the day. Pay attention to your urine color. Increase intake on training days and in hot weather. Replace electrolytes during long or intense sessions. These habits support performance, recovery, and long-term health.

Water is the most fundamental nutrient. Do not overlook it.

This chapter has provided you with the core nutritional principles that support longevity, metabolic health, and physical performance. These are not rigid rules. They are flexible guidelines that adapt to your life, your preferences, and your circumstances.

You now know that protein is the foundation. Aim for 1.6 to 2.2 grams per kilogram of body weight per day, distributed across three to four meals. Protein requirements increase with age due to anabolic resistance. Prioritize protein at every meal, and you will preserve muscle, support recovery, and maintain metabolic health.

You understand that carbohydrates are a tool, not an enemy. Match your carbohydrate intake to your activity level. Eat more on training days, less on rest days. Time carbohydrates around training sessions to support performance and recovery. Choose minimally processed sources high in fiber.

You know that fat is essential for hormone production, brain health, and satiety. Prioritize monounsaturated fats and omega-3s. Include moderate amounts of saturated fat from whole food sources. Avoid trans fats and excessive processed oils. Aim for 25 to 35 percent of total calories from fat.

You have learned that fiber is critical for metabolic health, gut health, blood sugar stability, and satiety. Aim for at least 25 to 38 grams per day from vegetables, fruits, whole grains, and legumes. Increase intake gradually to avoid digestive discomfort.

Finally, you understand that hydration is foundational. Drink water consistently throughout the day. Aim for 30 to 40 milliliters per kilogram of body weight, more on training days. Monitor your urine color and frequency. Replace electrolytes during long or intense training sessions.

These five principles, protein, carbohydrates, fat, fiber, and hydration, form the nutritional foundation of longevity. Master them, and the details take care of themselves. You do not need to count every calorie or track every macro forever. You just need to apply these principles consistently over time.

Before moving to Chapter 6, take a moment to assess your current nutrition. Are you eating enough protein? Are you matching carbohydrates to activity? Are you getting adequate healthy fats? Are you consuming enough fiber? Are you staying well-hydrated?

Identify one or two areas where you can improve immediately. Start there. Build from that foundation. Progress compounds over time.

Nutrition is not about perfection. It is about consistency. Apply these principles most of the time, and your body will respond with better energy, better performance, better body composition, and better long-term health.

CHAPTER 6: THE LONGEVITY PANTRY

Eating well begins long before you sit down to a meal. It begins in your kitchen, with the foods you keep on hand, the ingredients you stock, and the choices you make available to yourself.

If your pantry and refrigerator are filled with processed snacks, sugary cereals, and convenience foods, that is what you will eat, especially when you are tired, stressed, or short on time. If they are stocked with whole foods, quality proteins, and nutrient-dense ingredients, eating well becomes effortless.

This is the principle of environment design. You cannot rely on willpower alone. Willpower is a finite resource that depletes throughout the day. The easier you make it to eat well, the more likely you are to do it consistently. The harder you make it to eat poorly, the less often it will happen.

This chapter will guide you through building a longevity-focused pantry. You will learn which proteins to prioritize, which carbohydrates support metabolic health, which fats reduce inflammation, which herbs and spices boost nutrient intake, and which simple swaps make the biggest difference in real life.

This is not about perfection. You do not need to throw out everything in your kitchen and start from scratch. You do not need to buy expensive specialty foods or shop at multiple stores. You just need to gradually shift your pantry toward foods that support your goals.

Let's begin with the foundation: protein.

Essential Proteins

Protein should be the anchor of every meal, which means you need to keep a variety of high-quality protein sources readily available. The more options you have, the less likely you are to default to less optimal choices when you are hungry and short on time.

Eggs: Eggs are one of the most versatile, affordable, and nutritionally complete protein sources available. A large egg contains approximately 6 grams of protein along with healthy fats, vitamins A, D, E, and B12, choline, and antioxidants like lutein and zeaxanthin.

Keep a dozen or two in your refrigerator at all times. Eggs can be scrambled, fried, poached, hard-boiled, or added to dishes. Hard-boiled eggs make excellent grab-and-go snacks. Egg quality matters. Choose pasture-raised or omega-3 enriched eggs when possible. The nutritional profile is superior to conventional eggs.

Greek Yogurt and Cottage Cheese: Both are excellent high-protein dairy options. Greek yogurt contains approximately 15 to 20 grams of protein per cup, depending on the brand. Cottage cheese contains approximately 25 grams of protein per cup.

Choose full-fat or low-fat versions rather than fat-free. Fat-free versions often contain added sugars to compensate for flavor, and the fat helps with satiety and absorption of fat-soluble vitamins. Choose plain, unsweetened versions and add your own fruit, nuts, or a small amount of honey if desired.

These are perfect for breakfast, snacks, or post-workout meals. They pair well with berries, nuts, and seeds.

Chicken and Turkey: These lean poultry options are kitchen staples. Chicken breast contains approximately 30 grams of protein per 4-ounce serving with minimal fat. Chicken thighs contain slightly less protein but more fat, which makes them more flavorful and satisfying.

Buy both fresh and frozen. Frozen chicken is just as nutritious as fresh and allows you to keep protein on hand without worrying about spoilage. Rotisserie chickens are convenient for meal prep. Use the meat for salads, wraps, or quick meals, then use the bones to make bone broth.

Ground turkey is another versatile option. Use it in place of ground beef for a leaner alternative in dishes like chili, tacos, or meatballs.

Beef and Pork: Red meat provides not just protein but also highly bioavailable iron, zinc, and B vitamins. A 4-ounce serving of lean beef contains approximately 25 to 30 grams of protein.

Choose grass-fed beef when possible. It has a better omega-3 to omega-6 ratio and higher levels of conjugated linoleic acid (CLA), which may have health benefits. Leaner cuts like sirloin, tenderloin, and round minimize saturated fat intake. Fattier cuts like ribeye are fine occasionally but should not be your primary choice.

Pork tenderloin is one of the leanest cuts of meat available, comparable to chicken breast in fat content. Pork chops, ground pork, and pork shoulder are also versatile options.

Fish and Seafood: Fatty fish like salmon, sardines, mackerel, and trout are among the most nutrient-dense proteins available. They provide not just protein but also omega-3 fatty acids EPA and DHA, which support brain health, reduce inflammation, and protect cardiovascular function.

Aim for at least two servings of fatty fish per week. A 4-ounce serving of salmon contains approximately 25 grams of protein and up to 2 grams of omega-3s.

Keep canned or frozen fish on hand for convenience. Canned sardines, salmon, and tuna are shelf-stable, affordable, and just as nutritious as fresh. Choose options packed in water or olive oil rather than vegetable oil.

Shellfish like shrimp, scallops, and mussels are also excellent protein sources and cook quickly, making them ideal for weeknight meals.

Plant-Based Proteins: If you follow a plant-based diet or want to reduce animal protein consumption, keep these options stocked: tofu, tempeh, edamame, legumes (beans, lentils, chickpeas), and quinoa.

Tofu and tempeh are soy-based proteins that are highly versatile. Firm tofu contains approximately 10 grams of protein per half-cup and can be baked, stir-fried, or scrambled. Tempeh contains approximately 15 grams of protein per half-cup and has a firmer texture and nuttier flavor.

Legumes are among the most affordable protein sources available. One cup of cooked lentils contains approximately 18 grams of protein plus significant fiber. Keep dried and canned versions on hand. Canned beans are convenient for quick meals. Dried beans are more economical for meal prep.

Protein Powder: While whole food sources should be your priority, protein powder is a convenient option for meeting protein targets, especially post-workout or when traveling. Whey protein is the gold standard for muscle protein synthesis due to its high leucine content and rapid absorption. A typical serving contains 20 to 25 grams of protein.

Plant-based protein powders made from pea, rice, or hemp are also available. Choose versions with minimal added sugars and artificial ingredients. Look for products with at least 20 grams of protein per serving and a complete amino acid profile.

Deli Meats and Jerky: These are convenient options but should be consumed in moderation. Choose nitrate-free, minimally processed versions when possible. Look for products with recognizable ingredients and minimal added sugars.

Jerky, particularly beef or turkey jerky, makes an excellent portable snack. One ounce typically contains 9 to 12 grams of protein. Again, choose versions with minimal added sugars and avoid those with high sodium content.

Stocking your kitchen with a variety of these protein sources ensures you always have options available. Rotate through them to keep meals interesting and to ensure you are getting a diversity of nutrients.

Smart Carbohydrates

Not all carbohydrates are created equal. The quality of the carbohydrates you eat matters as much as the quantity. Prioritize whole, minimally processed sources that provide fiber, vitamins, minerals, and sustained energy without spiking blood sugar.

Vegetables (Non-Starchy): These should form the foundation of your carbohydrate intake. Leafy greens, cruciferous vegetables, peppers, tomatoes, cucumbers, zucchini, asparagus, and green beans are all low in calories and high in fiber, vitamins, minerals, and phytonutrients.

Keep fresh vegetables on hand and replenish them weekly. Frozen vegetables are just as nutritious as fresh and often more convenient. Keep bags of frozen broccoli, spinach, cauliflower, and mixed vegetables in your freezer for quick additions to any meal.

Aim to fill half your plate with non-starchy vegetables at lunch and dinner. They provide volume, fiber, and nutrients while keeping calorie density low.

Starchy Vegetables: Potatoes, sweet potatoes, butternut squash, and other starchy vegetables are nutrient-dense carbohydrate sources. A medium sweet potato contains approximately 25 grams of carbohydrates along with fiber, vitamin A, potassium, and antioxidants.

These are ideal for higher-carbohydrate days when you are training hard. They provide sustained energy without the blood sugar spike of refined carbohydrates. Leave the skin on when possible to maximize fiber intake.

Whole Grains: Oats, brown rice, quinoa, farro, barley, and whole wheat products provide carbohydrates along with fiber, B vitamins, and minerals. Choose minimally processed versions.

Oats are particularly valuable. One cup of cooked oats contains approximately 27 grams of carbohydrates and 4 grams of fiber. Oats are rich in beta-glucan, a type of soluble fiber that improves cholesterol and blood sugar control. Keep rolled oats or steel-cut oats in your pantry for quick, satisfying breakfasts.

Quinoa is a complete protein, meaning it contains all nine essential amino acids. One cup of cooked quinoa contains approximately 40 grams of carbohydrates and 8 grams of protein. It cooks quickly and is highly versatile.

Brown rice, while slower to cook, can be made in large batches and stored in the refrigerator for quick meals throughout the week.

Legumes: Beans, lentils, and chickpeas provide both carbohydrates and protein. One cup of cooked lentils contains approximately 40 grams of carbohydrates, 18 grams of protein, and 16 grams of fiber. This combination produces a very small blood sugar response despite the carbohydrate content.

Keep both canned and dried versions on hand. Canned legumes are convenient for adding to salads, soups, and quick meals. Dried legumes are more economical and allow you to control sodium content.

Fruits: Fruits provide carbohydrates along with fiber, vitamins, antioxidants, and phytonutrients. Berries (blueberries, strawberries, raspberries, blackberries) are particularly nutrient-dense and have a low glycemic impact due to their high fiber content.

Apples, pears, oranges, and bananas are convenient portable snacks. Bananas are particularly useful around training due to their easy digestibility and quick energy.

Keep fresh fruit on hand for snacks and to add to yogurt, oatmeal, or smoothies. Frozen berries are excellent for smoothies and can be kept on hand indefinitely.

Whole Grain Bread and Pasta: If you eat bread and pasta, choose whole grain versions. Look for products where the first ingredient is whole wheat flour or another whole grain, not enriched wheat flour. Check the fiber content: aim for at least 3 grams of fiber per serving for bread and at least 5 grams for pasta.

These are fine in moderation, particularly on training days, but should not be your primary carbohydrate sources. Vegetables, starchy vegetables, whole grains, and legumes should take priority.

Avoid or Minimize: White bread, white rice, pastries, sugary cereals, candy, soda, and most packaged snacks. These are refined carbohydrates that spike blood sugar, provide minimal nutrients, and contribute to insulin resistance when consumed regularly.

This does not mean you can never have them. It means they should be occasional treats, not daily staples. When you do choose them, consume them in the context of a meal with protein, fat, and fiber to blunt the blood sugar response.

Building your pantry around smart carbohydrates ensures that your default choices support stable blood sugar, sustained energy, and metabolic health.

Anti-Inflammatory Fats

The fats you choose have a profound impact on inflammation, hormone health, brain function, and cardiovascular health. Prioritize fats that reduce inflammation and support long-term health while minimizing those that promote inflammation.

Olive Oil: Extra virgin olive oil should be your primary cooking and salad oil. It is rich in monounsaturated fats and polyphenols, both of which reduce inflammation and support cardiovascular health. Studies consistently show that people who consume more olive oil have lower rates of heart disease, stroke, and all-cause mortality.

Choose extra virgin olive oil, which is less processed and retains more beneficial compounds than regular olive oil. Store it in a dark bottle away from heat and light to preserve quality. Use it for low to medium-heat cooking, salad dressings, and drizzling over finished dishes.

Avocado Oil: This is another excellent source of monounsaturated fats. It has a higher smoke point than olive oil, making it better for high-heat cooking. Use it for roasting, sautéing, or grilling.

Avocados: Whole avocados provide healthy fats along with fiber, potassium, and vitamins. Half an avocado contains approximately 15 grams of fat, mostly monounsaturated. Add avocado to salads, eggs, smoothies, or eat it on whole grain toast.

Nuts and Seeds: Almonds, walnuts, cashews, pecans, pumpkin seeds, chia seeds, and flaxseeds all provide healthy fats along with protein, fiber, and micronutrients.

Walnuts are particularly valuable because they are one of the richest plant sources of omega-3 fatty acids. One ounce of walnuts contains approximately 2.5 grams of omega-3s along with antioxidants and polyphenols.

Chia seeds and flaxseeds are also high in omega-3s. Add them to smoothies, oatmeal, or yogurt. Grind flaxseeds before consuming to maximize absorption.

Nuts and seeds are energy-dense, so pay attention to portions. A serving is typically one ounce, or about a small handful. Keep them in airtight containers or in the refrigerator to prevent rancidity.

Nut Butters: Almond butter, peanut butter, and other nut butters are convenient sources of healthy fats and protein. Choose natural versions with no added sugars or oils. The ingredient list should contain only nuts and possibly salt.

Fatty Fish: As discussed in the protein section, fatty fish like salmon, sardines, mackerel, and trout provide omega-3 fatty acids EPA and DHA. These are the most anti-inflammatory fats available and are critical for brain health, cardiovascular health, and reducing systemic inflammation.

If you do not eat fish regularly, consider supplementing with a high-quality fish oil. Look for products that provide at least 1,000 to 2,000 milligrams of combined EPA and DHA per serving and are third-party tested for purity.

Coconut Oil: Coconut oil is high in saturated fat, but it is primarily medium-chain triglycerides (MCTs), which are metabolized differently than long-chain saturated fats. Coconut oil has a high smoke point and is stable at high temperatures, making it suitable for cooking.

Use coconut oil in moderation. It is not a superfood, but it is a reasonable option for occasional use, particularly in baking or high-heat cooking.

Butter and Ghee: Butter from grass-fed cows contains higher levels of omega-3s and fat-soluble vitamins than conventional butter. Ghee, which is clarified butter, has the milk solids removed and is better tolerated by people with dairy sensitivities.

Use butter and ghee in moderation. They add flavor and satiety to meals but are high in saturated fat. A little goes a long way.

Avoid or Minimize: Processed vegetable oils like soybean, corn, sunflower, and safflower oil. These are high in omega-6 fatty acids, which promote inflammation when consumed in excess. Most packaged and fried foods contain these oils.

Also avoid trans fats, which are found in partially hydrogenated oils. Check ingredient labels and avoid any product that contains partially hydrogenated oil.

Stocking your kitchen with anti-inflammatory fats ensures that your default choices support long-term health rather than undermining it.

Herbs, Spices, and Micronutrient Boosters

Herbs and spices are often overlooked, but they are among the most nutrient-dense foods available. They provide antioxidants, anti-inflammatory compounds, and unique phytonutrients that support health in ways that go beyond basic nutrition.

Turmeric: Turmeric contains curcumin, a powerful anti-inflammatory compound. Chronic low-grade inflammation is at the root of most chronic diseases, and curcumin has been shown to reduce inflammatory markers. Combine turmeric with black pepper to enhance absorption. Use it in curries, soups, smoothies, or golden milk.

Ginger: Ginger has anti-inflammatory and digestive benefits. It can reduce nausea, improve digestion, and reduce muscle soreness after exercise. Use fresh ginger in stir-fries, teas, or smoothies, or keep ground ginger in your spice cabinet.

Garlic: Garlic contains allicin, a sulfur compound with antimicrobial and cardiovascular benefits. Regular garlic consumption is associated with lower blood pressure and improved cholesterol profiles. Use fresh garlic liberally in cooking.

Cinnamon: Cinnamon improves insulin sensitivity and helps regulate blood sugar. Studies show that consuming cinnamon with carbohydrate-rich meals reduces the post-meal blood sugar spike. Add cinnamon to oatmeal, yogurt, smoothies, or coffee.

Oregano, Rosemary, Thyme, and Basil: These herbs are rich in antioxidants and anti-inflammatory compounds. Use them fresh or dried to flavor meats, vegetables, and sauces.

Cayenne and Black Pepper: Both have metabolism-boosting properties. Cayenne contains capsaicin, which increases energy expenditure and fat oxidation. Black pepper contains piperine, which enhances the absorption of many nutrients, including curcumin from turmeric.

Sea Salt or Himalayan Salt: While excessive sodium intake is problematic, adequate sodium is necessary, especially if you train hard and sweat regularly. Use high-quality salt in moderation to season food. Avoid processed foods, which are the primary source of excess sodium in most diets.

Apple Cider Vinegar: Consuming vinegar with meals improves insulin sensitivity and reduces blood sugar spikes. One to two tablespoons of apple cider vinegar in water before meals or in salad dressings can be beneficial.

Dark Chocolate (70% or Higher): Dark chocolate is rich in antioxidants, particularly flavonoids, which support cardiovascular and cognitive health. Choose versions with at least seventy percent cocoa and minimal added sugar. A small square or two per day is sufficient.

Green Tea: Green tea contains catechins, particularly EGCG, which have antioxidant and metabolism-boosting properties. Drinking two to three cups per day is associated with improved fat oxidation, better cardiovascular health, and reduced risk of certain cancers.

Bone Broth: Bone broth is rich in collagen, gelatin, and amino acids like glycine and proline, which support gut health, joint health, and skin health. Make your own by simmering bones (chicken, beef, or fish) for twelve to twenty-four hours, or buy high-quality store-bought versions.

Keeping these herbs, spices, and micronutrient boosters in your pantry allows you to add flavor, variety, and health benefits to every meal without additional effort.

Simple Swaps for Real Life

You do not need to overhaul your entire diet overnight. Small, strategic swaps can have a significant impact over time. Here are practical substitutions that improve the nutritional quality of your meals without sacrificing satisfaction.

Instead of white rice → brown rice, quinoa, or cauliflower rice. Brown rice and quinoa provide more fiber and nutrients. Cauliflower rice is a low-carbohydrate option that adds volume without many calories.

Instead of white bread → whole grain bread or sourdough. Whole grain bread provides more fiber and produces a smaller blood sugar response. Sourdough, due to fermentation, has a lower glycemic index and is easier to digest.

Instead of sugary cereal → oatmeal, Greek yogurt, or eggs. These options provide sustained energy, more protein, and stable blood sugar without the sugar crash.

Instead of pasta → whole grain pasta, legume-based pasta, or zucchini noodles. Whole grain and legume-based pastas provide more fiber and protein. Zucchini noodles are a low-carbohydrate vegetable option.

Instead of chips → nuts, air-popped popcorn, or vegetable sticks with hummus. These options provide more nutrients and satiety without the empty calories and processed oils.

Instead of soda → sparkling water with lemon or lime, unsweetened iced tea, or water. Eliminating sugary drinks is one of the most impactful changes you can make for metabolic health.

Instead of creamy salad dressings → olive oil and vinegar, or make your own dressings. Most store-bought dressings contain processed oils and added sugars. Olive oil and vinegar is simple, healthy, and delicious.

Instead of fried foods → baked, grilled, or air-fried versions. You get similar textures and flavors without the excessive oil and calories.

Instead of candy and sweets → fresh fruit, dark chocolate, or a small portion of dried fruit. These options satisfy sweet cravings while providing nutrients and fiber.

Instead of processed snack bars → homemade energy balls, nuts, or fruit with nut butter. Most bars are highly processed with added sugars. Whole food options are more satisfying and nutritious.

Instead of fruit juice → whole fruit. Juice removes the fiber and concentrates the sugar, leading to blood sugar spikes. Whole fruit provides fiber, which slows absorption and increases satiety.

These swaps are not about deprivation. They are about upgrading the quality of what you eat while maintaining satisfaction. Over time, these small changes compound into significant improvements in energy, body composition, and metabolic health.

This chapter has given you the blueprint for building a longevity-focused pantry. You now know which proteins to keep on hand, which carbohydrates support metabolic health, which fats reduce inflammation, and which herbs and spices boost nutrient intake.

Stocking your kitchen with these foods is the most powerful step you can take toward eating well consistently. When your environment supports your goals, good choices become automatic. When you have to rely on willpower alone, you will eventually fail.

Before moving to the recipe section, take stock of your current pantry and refrigerator. What do you already have that aligns with these principles? What needs to be added? What should be removed or consumed less frequently?

Make a shopping list based on the categories in this chapter. Start with proteins, as they are the foundation of every meal. Add a variety of vegetables, both fresh and frozen. Include whole grains, legumes, and fruits. Stock healthy fats like olive oil, avocados, nuts, and seeds. Add herbs and spices to enhance flavor and nutrition.

You do not need to buy everything at once. Build your pantry gradually, replacing less optimal choices with better ones over time. Focus on progress, not perfection.

Remember, the goal is not to eat perfectly. The goal is to make the default choice the healthy choice. When eating well is easy and convenient, you will do it consistently. When it requires constant effort and decision-making, you will eventually revert to old patterns.

Design your environment to support your goals, and success becomes inevitable.

CHAPTER 7: BREAKFAST RECIPES

Breakfast sets the tone for your entire day. It is the first opportunity to provide your body with the nutrients it needs to function optimally, to stabilize blood sugar, and to support energy and focus for hours ahead.

Yet breakfast is often the meal people get wrong. They skip it entirely, grab a pastry and coffee on the way out the door, or pour a bowl of sugary cereal. These choices create blood sugar instability, energy crashes, and hunger that leads to poor decisions later in the day.

A longevity-focused breakfast is built around protein. It includes healthy fats for satiety and sustained energy. It provides fiber to stabilize blood sugar and support gut health. It is satisfying enough to keep you full for three to four hours without needing to snack.

This chapter provides ten breakfast recipes that meet these criteria. Each recipe includes preparation and cooking times, servings, macronutrient focus, blood sugar impact explanation, training-day pairing recommendations, substitutions for flexibility, and storage tips for meal prep.

These are not complicated recipes that require specialty ingredients or advanced cooking skills. They are practical, tested meals that fit into real life. Some can be prepared in minutes. Others can be made ahead in batches. All of them support your longevity goals.

Let's begin.

Recipe 1: Power Protein Scramble

Prep Time: 5 minutes
Cook Time: 8 minutes
Servings: 1

Ingredients:

- 3 large eggs

- 1 cup fresh spinach, roughly chopped

- ½ cup bell peppers, diced

- ¼ cup onion, diced

- 2 tablespoons feta cheese, crumbled

- 1 tablespoon olive oil

- Salt and black pepper to taste

- Optional: hot sauce for serving

Instructions:

1. Heat olive oil in a non-stick skillet over medium heat.

2. Add diced onions and bell peppers. Sauté for 3 to 4 minutes until softened.

3. Add chopped spinach and cook until wilted, about 1 minute.

4. In a small bowl, whisk the eggs with salt and pepper.

5. Pour eggs into the skillet with the vegetables. Let sit for 30 seconds, then gently scramble with a spatula, pulling the eggs from the edges toward the center.

6. When eggs are nearly set but still slightly glossy, remove from heat. The eggs will continue cooking from residual heat.

7. Top with crumbled feta cheese.

8. Serve immediately with optional hot sauce.

Macronutrient Focus: High protein (approximately 24 grams), moderate fat (approximately 22 grams), low carbohydrate (approximately 8 grams). This combination provides sustained energy without spiking blood sugar.

Blood Sugar Impact: Minimal. Eggs provide protein and fat with virtually no carbohydrates. The small amount of carbohydrates from vegetables and feta is offset by fiber and protein, resulting in a very stable blood sugar response. This meal will not cause an energy crash.

Best Training-Day Pairing: Excellent for any training day. The high protein supports muscle recovery. Eat this 1 to 2 hours before strength training for sustained energy, or immediately after training as part of recovery. On rest days, this is still an ideal choice for maintaining muscle and metabolic health.

Substitutions:

• Use any vegetables you have on hand: mushrooms, tomatoes, zucchini, or kale all work well.

• Replace feta with goat cheese, cheddar, or omit cheese entirely.

• Add cooked chicken sausage or turkey bacon for additional protein.

• Use egg whites only if you need to reduce fat intake, though whole eggs are more nutritious and satisfying.

Storage & Meal Prep Tips: You can pre-chop vegetables and store them in an airtight container in the refrigerator for up to 3 days, making morning prep faster. The scramble itself is best made fresh, but you can prepare it, let it cool, and store it in the refrigerator for up to 2 days. Reheat gently in a skillet or microwave. For meal prep, consider making a frittata version (see Recipe 2) which stores and reheats better than scrambled eggs.

Recipe 2: High-Protein Veggie Frittata

Prep Time: 10 minutes
Cook Time: 25 minutes
Servings: 4

Ingredients:

- 8 large eggs

- ½ cup milk (dairy or unsweetened almond milk)

- 1 cup broccoli florets, chopped small

- 1 cup cherry tomatoes, halved

- ½ cup red onion, diced

- 1 cup baby spinach

- ¾ cup shredded cheese (cheddar, mozzarella, or Gruyère)

- 2 tablespoons olive oil

- ½ teaspoon garlic powder

- Salt and black pepper to taste

- Fresh herbs (basil or parsley) for garnish

Instructions:

1. Preheat oven to 375°F (190°C).

2. Heat olive oil in a 10-inch oven-safe skillet over medium heat.

3. Add onion and broccoli. Sauté for 5 minutes until vegetables begin to soften.

4. Add spinach and cherry tomatoes. Cook for 2 minutes until spinach wilts.

5. In a large bowl, whisk together eggs, milk, garlic powder, salt, and pepper until well combined.

6. Pour egg mixture over the vegetables in the skillet, distributing evenly.

7. Sprinkle shredded cheese evenly over the top.

8. Transfer skillet to the oven and bake for 18 to 22 minutes, until the center is set and the edges are lightly golden. A knife inserted in the center should come out clean.

9. Remove from oven and let cool for 5 minutes before slicing.

10. Garnish with fresh herbs and serve.

Macronutrient Focus: High protein (approximately 18 grams per serving), moderate fat (approximately 16 grams), low carbohydrate (approximately 6 grams). The vegetables add fiber and micronutrients without significantly impacting blood sugar.

Blood Sugar Impact: Minimal to none. This is a low-glycemic meal that provides steady energy for 3 to 4 hours. The combination of protein, fat, and fiber from vegetables produces virtually no blood sugar spike.

Best Training-Day Pairing: Perfect for any day. The high protein makes this ideal for post-strength training recovery. It is also excellent for rest days as it maintains muscle without excess carbohydrates. Pair with a piece of fruit or whole grain toast on heavy training days if you need additional carbohydrates.

Substitutions:

- Use any combination of vegetables: mushrooms, zucchini, asparagus, bell peppers, or kale.

- Swap cheese for a dairy-free alternative if needed.

- Add cooked ground turkey, chicken sausage, or crumbled bacon for additional protein and flavor.

- Use egg whites only for a lower-fat version, though this reduces satiety.

Storage & Meal Prep Tips: Frittatas are excellent for meal prep. Let the frittata cool completely, then cut into 4 wedges. Store in individual airtight containers in the refrigerator for up to 4 days. Reheat in the microwave for 60 to 90 seconds or in a 350°F oven for 10 minutes. You can also freeze individual portions wrapped in plastic wrap and foil for up to 2 months. Thaw overnight in the refrigerator before reheating.

Recipe 3: Greek Yogurt Power Bowl

Prep Time: 5 minutes
Cook Time: 0 minutes
Servings: 1

Ingredients:

- 1 cup plain Greek yogurt (full-fat or 2%)

- ¼ cup mixed berries (blueberries, strawberries, raspberries)

- 2 tablespoons chopped walnuts or almonds

- 1 tablespoon ground flaxseed

- 1 tablespoon chia seeds

- ½ teaspoon cinnamon

- Optional: 1 teaspoon raw honey or a few drops of stevia

Instructions:

1. Place Greek yogurt in a bowl.

2. Top with mixed berries.

3. Sprinkle with chopped nuts, ground flaxseed, and chia seeds.

4. Dust with cinnamon.

5. Drizzle with honey if using.

6. Mix together or eat in layers.

Macronutrient Focus: High protein (approximately 25 grams), moderate fat (approximately 14 grams), moderate carbohydrate (approximately 25 grams). The carbohydrates come primarily from berries and are offset by significant protein, fat, and fiber.

Blood Sugar Impact: Low to moderate. Greek yogurt is high in protein, which blunts blood sugar response. Berries are among the lowest-glycemic fruits due to their high fiber content. The nuts, seeds, and healthy fats further slow digestion and glucose absorption. This meal produces a gentle, sustained rise in blood sugar without a crash.

Best Training-Day Pairing: Excellent for rest days or light activity days. The moderate carbohydrate content from berries provides some fuel without excess. This is also a good post-workout option after Zone 2 cardio or mobility work. For heavy strength training days, add a banana or additional berries to increase carbohydrate intake.

Substitutions:

- Use any type of berries or mix with diced apple or pear.

- Replace walnuts with pecans, cashews, or sunflower seeds.

- Add a scoop of protein powder to increase protein content to 45+ grams.

- Use coconut yogurt for a dairy-free version, though protein content will be lower unless you add protein powder.

- Swap chia seeds for hemp seeds or additional flaxseed.

Storage & Meal Prep Tips: This bowl is best assembled fresh, but you can prep components in advance. Portion Greek yogurt into containers for the week. Pre-measure nuts, seeds, and berries into small bags or containers. In the morning, simply combine. If making the night before, keep berries separate and add just before eating to prevent them from making the yogurt watery. The assembled bowl can be stored in the refrigerator for up to 2 days.

Recipe 4: Savory Oatmeal with Egg

Prep Time: 5 minutes
Cook Time: 12 minutes
Servings: 1

Ingredients:

- ½ cup rolled oats

- 1 cup low-sodium chicken or vegetable broth

- 1 large egg

- ½ cup fresh spinach or kale, chopped

- ¼ avocado, sliced

- 1 tablespoon grated Parmesan cheese

- 1 teaspoon olive oil

- Salt, black pepper, and red pepper flakes to taste

- Optional: 1 tablespoon chopped green onions

Instructions:

1. In a small pot, bring broth to a boil.

2. Add oats and reduce heat to medium-low. Simmer for 7 to 10 minutes, stirring occasionally, until oats are tender and have absorbed most of the liquid.

3. Stir in chopped spinach or kale and cook for 1 minute until wilted.

4. Season with salt and black pepper.

5. Transfer oatmeal to a bowl.

6. In a small skillet, heat olive oil over medium heat. Fry the egg to your preference (over easy or sunny side up works best).

7. Top the savory oatmeal with the fried egg, avocado slices, Parmesan cheese, and optional green onions.

8. Season with additional black pepper and red pepper flakes if desired.

Macronutrient Focus: High protein (approximately 16 grams), moderate fat (approximately 18 grams), moderate carbohydrate (approximately 32 grams). The carbohydrates from oats provide sustained energy, while protein and fat create satiety.

Blood Sugar Impact: Low to moderate. Oats contain beta-glucan, a type of soluble fiber that slows glucose absorption and improves insulin sensitivity. Cooking oats in broth rather than water does not impact blood sugar. The addition of egg, avocado, and cheese provides protein and fat that further stabilizes blood sugar response. This meal provides steady energy for 3 to 4 hours.

Best Training-Day Pairing: Ideal for moderate to high training days, particularly before Zone 2 cardio or lighter strength sessions. The carbohydrates from oats provide readily available energy without being excessive. This is also excellent 1 to 2 hours before a morning workout. On rest days, reduce the oat portion to ⅓ cup.

Substitutions:

- Use steel-cut oats for a chewier texture (increase cooking time to 20 minutes).

- Replace spinach with arugula, Swiss chard, or any leafy green.

- Use feta or goat cheese instead of Parmesan.

- Add sautéed mushrooms for additional flavor and nutrients.
- Replace the egg with grilled chicken or turkey sausage for variety.

Storage & Meal Prep Tips: Cook oats in broth ahead of time and store in the refrigerator for up to 4 days. Reheat individual portions in the microwave with a splash of additional broth to restore creaminess. Cook the egg fresh each morning. You can pre-chop vegetables and store them in containers for quick assembly. This meal is best assembled fresh but can be mostly prepped in advance.

Recipe 5: Protein-Packed Smoothie

Prep Time: 5 minutes
Cook Time: 0 minutes
Servings: 1

Ingredients:

- 1 scoop vanilla or unflavored protein powder (whey or plant-based, approximately 20-25g protein)
- 1 cup unsweetened almond milk or milk of choice
- ½ cup frozen mixed berries
- ½ banana (fresh or frozen)
- 1 tablespoon almond butter or peanut butter
- 1 tablespoon ground flaxseed
- 1 cup fresh spinach or kale
- ½ teaspoon cinnamon
- Ice cubes as needed
- Optional: ¼ teaspoon vanilla extract

Instructions:

1. Add all ingredients to a high-speed blender in the order listed (liquid first helps blending).
2. Blend on high for 45 to 60 seconds until completely smooth.
3. Check consistency. If too thick, add more liquid. If too thin, add ice or more frozen fruit.
4. Pour into a glass and consume immediately.

Macronutrient Focus: High protein (approximately 30 grams), moderate fat (approximately 12 grams), moderate carbohydrate (approximately 35 grams). This is a complete meal in liquid form.

Blood Sugar Impact: Low to moderate. The protein powder and nut butter provide substantial protein and fat that slow the absorption of carbohydrates from fruit. The fiber from berries, banana, flaxseed, and greens further stabilizes blood sugar. The glycemic impact is much lower than drinking fruit juice. This smoothie provides steady energy without a crash.

Best Training-Day Pairing: Excellent for post-workout recovery, particularly after strength training or high-intensity intervals. The combination of protein and carbohydrates supports muscle recovery and glycogen replenishment. Also suitable for busy mornings when you need a quick, complete meal. On rest days, reduce or eliminate the banana to lower carbohydrate content.

Substitutions:

- Use any frozen fruit: mango, pineapple, cherries, or peaches.

- Replace nut butter with ¼ avocado for healthy fats.

- Add a handful of oats for additional carbohydrates on heavy training days.

- Use full-fat Greek yogurt instead of protein powder for a creamier texture (adjust liquid as needed).

- Add collagen peptides for additional protein and joint support.

- Include 1 teaspoon of spirulina or chlorella for added micronutrients (optional).

Storage & Meal Prep Tips: Smoothies are best consumed immediately, but you can prep freezer packs for quick blending. Place all ingredients except liquid and protein powder into individual freezer bags or containers. In the morning, dump the frozen contents into the blender, add liquid and protein powder, and blend. Smoothies can be stored in the refrigerator for up to 24 hours in an airtight container. Shake or stir before drinking as separation is normal. For best texture, blend fresh each time.

Recipe 6: Almond Flour Protein Pancakes

Prep Time: 5 minutes
Cook Time: 10 minutes
Servings: 2 (approximately 6 small pancakes)

Ingredients:

- 1 cup almond flour

- 2 large eggs

- 2 tablespoons unsweetened almond milk

- 1 scoop vanilla protein powder (optional, for higher protein)

- 1 teaspoon baking powder

- ½ teaspoon cinnamon

- ¼ teaspoon vanilla extract

- Pinch of salt

- Coconut oil or butter for cooking

- Toppings: fresh berries, Greek yogurt, almond butter, or sugar-free maple syrup

Instructions:

1. In a medium bowl, whisk together almond flour, protein powder (if using), baking powder, cinnamon, and salt.

2. In a separate small bowl, whisk together eggs, almond milk, and vanilla extract.

3. Pour wet ingredients into dry ingredients and mix until just combined. The batter will be thick. Let sit for 2 minutes to allow almond flour to absorb liquid.

4. Heat a non-stick skillet or griddle over medium-low heat. Add a small amount of coconut oil or butter.

5. Pour approximately ¼ cup of batter per pancake onto the skillet. Use the back of a spoon to gently spread into a circle.

6. Cook for 2 to 3 minutes until bubbles form on the surface and edges begin to set.

7. Flip carefully and cook for another 2 minutes until golden brown.

8. Repeat with remaining batter, adding more oil as needed.

9. Serve warm with desired toppings.

Macronutrient Focus: High protein (approximately 20 grams per serving without protein powder, 30+ grams with), high fat (approximately 28 grams), low carbohydrate (approximately 12 grams). Almond flour is naturally low in carbohydrates and high in healthy fats.

Blood Sugar Impact: Minimal. Almond flour has a very low glycemic index compared to wheat flour. The high protein and fat content creates sustained energy without blood sugar spikes. Even with toppings like berries, the blood sugar response remains moderate and stable.

Best Training-Day Pairing: Suitable for any day. The lower carbohydrate content makes these ideal for rest days or light activity days. For heavy training days, pair with a banana, additional berries, or a small amount of honey or maple syrup to increase carbohydrates. Also excellent post-workout when topped with Greek yogurt for additional protein.

Substitutions:

- Replace almond flour with coconut flour (use ⅓ cup coconut flour and increase eggs to 4, as coconut flour is more absorbent).

- Use whole wheat flour for a more traditional pancake with higher carbohydrates.

- Replace almond milk with any milk of choice.

- Add ½ mashed banana to the batter for natural sweetness and additional carbohydrates.

- Mix in dark chocolate chips or blueberries for variety.

Storage & Meal Prep Tips: These pancakes are excellent for meal prep. Let pancakes cool completely, then layer between sheets of parchment paper and store in an airtight container or freezer bag. Refrigerate for up to 4 days or freeze for up to 2 months. Reheat in a toaster, toaster oven, or microwave. Frozen pancakes can be reheated directly from the freezer. Make a large batch on Sunday to have quick breakfasts throughout the week.

Recipe 7: Cottage Cheese and Avocado Toast

Prep Time: 5 minutes
Cook Time: 2 minutes
Servings: 1

Ingredients:

- 2 slices whole grain bread or sourdough

- ½ cup cottage cheese (full-fat or low-fat)

- ½ avocado, mashed

- 1 large egg (optional, for additional protein)

- Everything bagel seasoning or red pepper flakes

- Salt and black pepper to taste

- Optional: cherry tomatoes, cucumber slices, or microgreens for topping

Instructions:

1. Toast bread to desired doneness.

2. While bread is toasting, mash avocado in a small bowl with a fork. Season with salt and pepper.

3. If using an egg, fry or poach it to your preference.

4. Spread cottage cheese evenly on one slice of toast.

5. Spread mashed avocado on the other slice.

6. Top cottage cheese toast with the egg (if using) and everything bagel seasoning.

7. Top avocado toast with optional cherry tomatoes, cucumber, or microgreens, and season with red pepper flakes.

8. Serve immediately.

Macronutrient Focus: High protein (approximately 28 grams with egg, 22 grams without), moderate fat (approximately 20 grams), moderate carbohydrate (approximately 30 grams). The protein from cottage cheese and egg creates significant satiety.

Blood Sugar Impact: Low to moderate. Whole grain bread provides fiber that slows glucose absorption. The high protein from cottage cheese and egg, combined with healthy fats from avocado, significantly blunts blood sugar response. This meal provides steady energy for 3 to 4 hours without a crash.

Best Training-Day Pairing: Suitable for moderate training days or 1 to 2 hours before morning training. The carbohydrates from bread provide readily available energy. Also excellent for post-Zone 2 cardio or light strength sessions. On rest days, use one slice of bread instead of two to reduce carbohydrate intake.

Substitutions:

- Use gluten-free bread if needed.

- Replace cottage cheese with ricotta cheese or Greek yogurt.

- Use smoked salmon instead of an egg for omega-3s and different flavor.

- Add hemp seeds or pumpkin seeds for additional healthy fats and protein.

- Replace avocado with hummus for a different fat source.

Storage & Meal Prep Tips: This meal is best assembled fresh. However, you can prep components in advance. Pre-mash avocado and store in an airtight container with a squeeze of lemon juice to prevent browning (refrigerate for up to 1 day). Hard-boil eggs in advance and store in the refrigerator for up to 5 days. Toast and assemble each morning for best texture. Avoid assembling the night before, as bread will become soggy.

Recipe 8: Breakfast Burrito Bowl

Prep Time: 5 minutes
Cook Time: 10 minutes
Servings: 1

Ingredients:

- 2 large eggs

- ¼ cup black beans, drained and rinsed

- ½ cup cooked brown rice or quinoa

- ¼ cup diced bell peppers

- ¼ cup diced tomatoes

- ¼ avocado, sliced

- 2 tablespoons shredded cheddar or Mexican blend cheese

- 1 tablespoon salsa

- 1 tablespoon Greek yogurt or sour cream

- 1 teaspoon olive oil

- Salt, black pepper, and cumin to taste

- Optional: hot sauce, cilantro, lime wedge

Instructions:

1. Heat olive oil in a skillet over medium heat.

2. Add diced bell peppers and cook for 2 to 3 minutes until softened.

3. Add black beans and cooked rice or quinoa. Season with cumin, salt, and pepper. Cook for 2 minutes until heated through.

4. Transfer bean and rice mixture to a bowl.

5. In the same skillet, scramble or fry eggs to your preference.

6. Place eggs on top of the bean and rice mixture.

7. Top with diced tomatoes, avocado slices, shredded cheese, salsa, and Greek yogurt.

8. Garnish with optional cilantro and a squeeze of lime. Add hot sauce if desired.

Macronutrient Focus: High protein (approximately 24 grams), moderate fat (approximately 18 grams), moderate carbohydrate (approximately 42 grams). This is a balanced meal with carbohydrates from beans and rice, protein from eggs and beans, and healthy fats from avocado.

Blood Sugar Impact: Low to moderate. Black beans are high in fiber and protein, which significantly slow glucose absorption. The combination of protein, fat, and fiber creates a gentle, sustained blood sugar response. This meal provides energy for 3 to 4 hours.

Best Training-Day Pairing: Excellent for moderate to high training days. The carbohydrates from beans and rice provide fuel for strength training or cardio. This is ideal 1 to 2 hours before training or as a post-workout recovery meal. On rest days, reduce rice to ¼ cup or eliminate it entirely.

Substitutions:

- Use pinto beans, kidney beans, or refried beans instead of black beans.

- Replace rice with cauliflower rice for a lower-carbohydrate version.

- Use sweet potato cubes instead of rice for a different carbohydrate source.

- Add cooked ground turkey or chicken for additional protein.

- Replace Greek yogurt with full sour cream or omit if dairy-free.

- Use dairy-free cheese or nutritional yeast for a vegan version (replace eggs with scrambled tofu).

Storage & Meal Prep Tips: This bowl is excellent for meal prep. Cook rice and beans in bulk at the beginning of the week. Store in separate containers in the refrigerator for up to 5 days. Pre-chop vegetables and store in containers. Each morning, reheat the base ingredients and cook eggs fresh for best texture. You can also assemble complete bowls without eggs, refrigerate for up to 3 days, and add a freshly cooked egg when ready to eat. Avoid adding avocado, salsa, and Greek yogurt until serving.

Recipe 9: Smoked Salmon and Cream Cheese Plate

Prep Time: 5 minutes
Cook Time: 0 minutes
Servings: 1

Ingredients:

- 3 ounces smoked salmon

- 2 tablespoons cream cheese (full-fat or low-fat)

- ½ cup cherry tomatoes, halved

- ½ cup cucumber slices

- ¼ red onion, thinly sliced

- 1 tablespoon capers

- 1 hard-boiled egg, sliced (optional for additional protein)

- Fresh dill for garnish

- Lemon wedge

- Optional: 1 slice whole grain bread or crackers

Instructions:

1. Arrange smoked salmon on a plate.

2. Add dollops of cream cheese alongside the salmon.

3. Arrange cherry tomatoes, cucumber slices, red onion, and capers on the plate.

4. Add sliced hard-boiled egg if using.

5. Garnish with fresh dill.

6. Serve with a lemon wedge for squeezing over the salmon.

7. If using bread or crackers, serve on the side.

Macronutrient Focus: High protein (approximately 26 grams with egg, 20 grams without), moderate fat (approximately 14 grams), low carbohydrate (approximately 8 grams without bread). This is a protein and fat-focused meal with minimal carbohydrates.

Blood Sugar Impact: Minimal to none. Smoked salmon provides protein and omega-3 fatty acids with no carbohydrates. Cream cheese adds fat and minimal carbohydrates. Vegetables provide fiber. This meal has virtually no impact on blood sugar and provides sustained energy.

Best Training-Day Pairing: Ideal for rest days or light activity days due to low carbohydrate content. Also excellent for post-Zone 2 cardio when carbohydrate needs are moderate. For heavy training days, add whole grain bread or crackers to increase carbohydrates. The omega-3s from salmon support recovery and reduce inflammation, making this suitable any time.

Substitutions:

- Replace smoked salmon with cooked salmon, grilled chicken, or hard-boiled eggs.

- Use goat cheese or ricotta instead of cream cheese.

- Add avocado slices for additional healthy fats.

- Include olives for additional flavor and healthy fats.

- Use bell pepper slices or celery instead of cucumber.

- Add Everything bagel seasoning for additional flavor.

Storage & Meal Prep Tips: This plate is best assembled fresh, but components can be prepped in advance. Hard-boil eggs and store in the refrigerator for up to 5 days. Pre-slice vegetables and store in airtight containers for up to 3 days. Keep smoked salmon in its original packaging or transfer to an airtight container and refrigerate. Assemble the plate each morning for best freshness. This meal is ideal for busy mornings because it requires no cooking.

Recipe 10: Sweet Potato and Egg Hash

Prep Time: 8 minutes
Cook Time: 15 minutes
Servings: 2

Ingredients:

- 1 large sweet potato, peeled and diced small (approximately 2 cups)

- 4 large eggs

- ½ cup diced onion

- ½ cup diced bell pepper (any color)

- 2 cups fresh spinach or kale, chopped

- 2 tablespoons olive oil or avocado oil

- 1 teaspoon smoked paprika

- ½ teaspoon garlic powder

- Salt and black pepper to taste

- Optional: hot sauce, avocado slices, or salsa for serving

Instructions:

1. Heat 1 tablespoon of oil in a large skillet over medium heat.

2. Add diced sweet potato and season with smoked paprika, garlic powder, salt, and pepper.

3. Cook for 10 to 12 minutes, stirring occasionally, until sweet potatoes are tender and beginning to brown. If they start to stick, add a splash of water.

4. Add diced onion and bell pepper. Cook for 3 to 4 minutes until softened.

5. Add chopped spinach or kale and cook for 1 minute until wilted.

6. Push the hash to the sides of the skillet, creating four wells in the center.

7. Add remaining 1 tablespoon of oil to the center and crack eggs into the wells.

8. Cover the skillet and cook for 3 to 5 minutes until eggs are cooked to your preference.

9. Season eggs with additional salt and pepper.

10. Serve immediately with optional toppings.

Macronutrient Focus: High protein (approximately 14 grams per serving), moderate fat (approximately 16 grams), moderate to high carbohydrate (approximately 28 grams). The carbohydrates from sweet potato provide sustained energy, especially valuable for training days.

Blood Sugar Impact: Low to moderate. Sweet potatoes have a lower glycemic index than white potatoes due to their fiber content. The protein and fat from eggs, combined with fiber from vegetables, create a balanced blood sugar response. This meal provides steady energy for 3 to 4 hours without a crash.

Best Training-Day Pairing: Excellent for moderate to high training days, particularly before morning strength training sessions. The carbohydrates from sweet potato provide readily available fuel. Also suitable as a post-workout meal to replenish glycogen. On rest days, reduce sweet potato to ½ cup per serving.

Substitutions:

- Replace sweet potato with white potato, butternut squash, or additional vegetables for lower carbohydrates.

- Use any combination of vegetables: mushrooms, zucchini, tomatoes, or broccoli.

- Add cooked ground turkey, chicken sausage, or bacon for additional protein and flavor.

- Use egg whites only if reducing fat intake, though whole eggs are more nutritious.

- Season with different spices: cumin, chili powder, or Italian seasoning.

Storage & Meal Prep Tips: This hash is excellent for meal prep. Cook the sweet potato and vegetable mixture in bulk, let cool, and store in airtight containers in the refrigerator for up to 4 days. Each morning, reheat a portion in a skillet and add a freshly cooked egg, or cook eggs separately and add to the reheated hash. You can also prepare complete servings with eggs, refrigerate for up to 3 days, and reheat in the microwave (though eggs may be slightly rubbery when reheated). For best texture, cook eggs fresh each day.

These ten breakfast recipes provide variety, flexibility, and nutritional balance to start your day optimally. Each recipe prioritizes protein, includes healthy fats, and incorporates fiber from vegetables or whole grains. They are designed to stabilize blood sugar, support muscle maintenance, and provide sustained energy without mid-morning crashes.

The recipes range from quick no-cook options like the Greek Yogurt Power Bowl and Smoked Salmon Plate to slightly more involved preparations like the High-Protein Veggie Frittata and Sweet Potato Hash. Several recipes are ideal for meal prep, allowing you to prepare breakfast components in advance and assemble quickly during busy mornings.

Remember that these recipes are templates, not rigid prescriptions. Adjust portion sizes based on your body size, activity level, and training schedule. Substitute ingredients based on preferences, dietary restrictions, or what you have available. The principles remain the same: prioritize protein, include healthy fats, choose quality carbohydrates, and add vegetables whenever possible.

As you incorporate these breakfasts into your routine, pay attention to how they make you feel. Do they keep you satisfied for 3 to 4 hours? Do you have steady energy, or do you crash before lunch? Do you feel mentally clear and focused? Use this feedback to adjust portions and macronutrient ratios to match your individual needs.

Breakfast is not just about eating. It is about setting yourself up for success for the entire day. When you start with a protein-rich, blood-sugar-stabilizing meal, you make better decisions throughout the day. You have more energy for training. You recover better. You maintain muscle mass and metabolic health.

Make breakfast a priority, not an afterthought. Your body will thank you for decades.

Lunch is where many people lose their nutritional discipline. The morning starts well, but by midday, hunger strikes, time is short, and convenient options beckon. A trip to the drive-through, a vending machine snack, or skipping lunch entirely become the default.

This pattern creates problems. Skipping lunch leads to excessive hunger later, which drives poor dinner choices and evening snacking. Choosing convenience foods, which are typically high in refined carbohydrates and low in protein, creates blood sugar instability, afternoon energy crashes, and undermines your training and recovery.

A well-constructed lunch should accomplish several things: it should provide adequate protein to support muscle maintenance and satiety, include vegetables for fiber and micronutrients, contain appropriate carbohydrates based on your training schedule, and keep you satisfied for four to five hours without an energy crash.

This chapter provides twelve lunch recipes that meet these criteria. They range from quick salads and wraps that can be assembled in minutes to heartier bowls and soups that can be prepared in batches for the week. Each recipe includes the same detailed information as the breakfast chapter: timing, servings, macronutrient focus, blood sugar impact, training-day pairing, substitutions, and meal prep guidance.

These recipes are designed for real life. They accommodate busy schedules, limited cooking skills, and the need for portability. Many can be packed in containers and taken to work. Others can be prepared on Sunday and eaten throughout the week.

Let's begin.

Recipe 1: Mediterranean Chicken Bowl

Prep Time: 10 minutes
Cook Time: 15 minutes
Servings: 2

Ingredients:

- 12 ounces chicken breast, diced

- 2 cups mixed greens or baby spinach

- 1 cup cherry tomatoes, halved

- 1 cucumber, diced

- ½ cup Kalamata olives, pitted and halved

- ½ cup red onion, thinly sliced

- ½ cup crumbled feta cheese

- ¼ cup hummus

- 2 tablespoons olive oil

- 1 tablespoon lemon juice

- 1 teaspoon dried oregano

- 1 teaspoon garlic powder

- Salt and black pepper to taste

- Optional: ½ cup cooked quinoa or brown rice per serving

Instructions:

1. Season diced chicken with oregano, garlic powder, salt, and pepper.

2. Heat 1 tablespoon of olive oil in a skillet over medium-high heat.

3. Add chicken and cook for 6 to 8 minutes, stirring occasionally, until cooked through and lightly browned. Remove from heat.

4. In a small bowl, whisk together remaining 1 tablespoon of olive oil, lemon juice, salt, and pepper to make a simple dressing.

5. Divide mixed greens between two bowls.

6. Top each bowl with cooked chicken, cherry tomatoes, cucumber, olives, red onion, and crumbled feta.

7. Add a dollop of hummus to each bowl.

8. Drizzle with lemon-olive oil dressing.

9. If using, add cooked quinoa or brown rice to each bowl.

10. Toss before eating or eat in layers.

Macronutrient Focus: High protein (approximately 38 grams without grains, 42 grams with), moderate fat (approximately 22 grams), low to moderate carbohydrate (approximately 18 grams without grains, 38 grams with). This is a protein-focused meal with healthy Mediterranean fats.

Blood Sugar Impact: Minimal without grains, low to moderate with grains. The high protein from chicken, combined with healthy fats from olive oil, olives, and feta, creates excellent blood sugar stability. Vegetables provide fiber without significant carbohydrates. Adding quinoa or rice increases carbohydrates but remains balanced due to the high protein and fat content.

Best Training-Day Pairing: Without grains, this is ideal for rest days or light activity days. With quinoa or rice added, it becomes excellent for moderate to high training days, particularly after strength training or as a pre-training meal 2 to 3 hours before exercise. The Mediterranean fats support hormone health and reduce inflammation.

Substitutions:

- Replace chicken with grilled shrimp, salmon, or chickpeas for a vegetarian version.

- Use goat cheese or omit cheese entirely for dairy-free.

- Replace hummus with tahini dressing or avocado.

- Add roasted red peppers or artichoke hearts for additional flavor.

- Use romaine lettuce or arugula instead of mixed greens.

- Replace olives with sun-dried tomatoes if you prefer.

Storage & Meal Prep Tips: This bowl is excellent for meal prep. Cook chicken in bulk and store in the refrigerator for up to 4 days. Prep all vegetables and store in separate containers. Store dressing separately. Assemble bowls each day for best texture, or assemble complete bowls without dressing and store in the refrigerator for up to 3 days. Add dressing just before eating to prevent wilting. If including grains, cook in bulk and store separately, adding to bowls as needed.

Recipe 2: Turkey and Avocado Wrap

Prep Time: 8 minutes
Cook Time: 0 minutes
Servings: 1

Ingredients:

- 1 large whole wheat or spinach tortilla (10-inch)

- 4 ounces sliced turkey breast (deli or leftover roasted turkey)

- ½ avocado, sliced

- ¼ cup shredded carrots

- ¼ cup shredded red cabbage

- ¼ cup sliced cucumber

- 2 tablespoons hummus or Greek yogurt

- 1 cup mixed greens or spinach

- 1 tablespoon Dijon mustard or hot sauce

- Salt and black pepper to taste

Instructions:

1. Lay the tortilla flat on a clean surface.

2. Spread hummus or Greek yogurt evenly over the center of the tortilla, leaving about 1 inch around the edges.

3. Add a thin layer of Dijon mustard or a few dashes of hot sauce if using.

4. Layer turkey slices in the center of the tortilla.

5. Top with avocado slices, shredded carrots, cabbage, cucumber, and mixed greens.

6. Season with salt and black pepper.

7. Fold in the sides of the tortilla, then roll tightly from bottom to top, tucking in the filling as you go.

8. Cut in half diagonally.

9. Serve immediately or wrap tightly in foil or plastic wrap for transport.

Macronutrient Focus: High protein (approximately 32 grams), moderate fat (approximately 18 grams), moderate carbohydrate (approximately 35 grams). This is a balanced, portable meal with substantial protein for satiety.

Blood Sugar Impact: Low to moderate. Whole wheat tortilla provides fiber that slows glucose absorption. The high protein from turkey, combined with healthy fats from avocado, creates a balanced blood sugar response. Vegetables add additional fiber. This wrap provides sustained energy for 4 to 5 hours.

Best Training-Day Pairing: Suitable for moderate training days. The carbohydrates from the tortilla provide energy without being excessive. This is an excellent post-Zone 2 cardio meal or 2 to 3 hours before afternoon training. On rest days, use a low-carb tortilla or lettuce wraps instead.

Substitutions:

- Replace turkey with chicken, roast beef, or hard-boiled eggs.

- Use a low-carb tortilla, collard green wrap, or large lettuce leaves for lower carbohydrate content.

- Replace avocado with roasted red peppers or additional hummus.

- Add sprouts, tomatoes, or bell peppers for variety.

- Use mustard, tahini, or balsamic vinegar instead of hummus.

- For a vegetarian version, use chickpeas, tempeh, or additional vegetables.

Storage & Meal Prep Tips: Wraps are best assembled fresh for optimal texture, but you can prep components in advance. Pre-cook and slice protein, wash and chop vegetables, and store in separate containers. Assemble wraps each morning. If you must assemble the night before, wrap tightly in plastic wrap or foil and refrigerate. Keep wet ingredients like tomatoes separate and add before eating to prevent sogginess. Wraps can be stored assembled for up to 24 hours in the refrigerator.

Recipe 3: Tuna and White Bean Salad

Prep Time: 10 minutes
Cook Time: 0 minutes
Servings: 2

Ingredients:

- 2 cans (5 ounces each) tuna in water, drained

- 1 can (15 ounces) white beans (cannellini or great northern), drained and rinsed

- 2 cups arugula or mixed greens

- 1 cup cherry tomatoes, halved

- ½ red onion, thinly sliced

- ¼ cup fresh parsley, chopped

- 3 tablespoons olive oil

- 2 tablespoons lemon juice

- 1 teaspoon Dijon mustard

- 1 garlic clove, minced

- Salt and black pepper to taste

- Optional: ¼ cup crumbled feta cheese

Instructions:

1. In a large bowl, combine drained tuna and white beans.

2. Add arugula, cherry tomatoes, red onion, and parsley.

3. In a small bowl, whisk together olive oil, lemon juice, Dijon mustard, minced garlic, salt, and pepper to create the dressing.

4. Pour dressing over the salad and toss gently to combine.

5. Divide between two bowls or plates.

6. Top with optional crumbled feta cheese.

7. Serve immediately or refrigerate for up to 2 hours before serving.

Macronutrient Focus: High protein (approximately 35 grams), moderate fat (approximately 16 grams), moderate carbohydrate (approximately 28 grams). White beans provide both protein and carbohydrates along with significant fiber.

Blood Sugar Impact: Low to moderate. White beans are high in fiber and protein, which significantly slow glucose absorption. The glycemic impact is very low despite the carbohydrate content. Combined with protein from tuna and healthy fats from olive oil, this meal produces stable, sustained energy.

Best Training-Day Pairing: Excellent for moderate training days or as a post-workout meal after Zone 2 cardio or lighter strength training. The carbohydrates from beans support glycogen replenishment without being excessive. Also suitable for rest days due to the balanced macronutrient profile. The omega-3s from tuna support recovery and reduce inflammation.

Substitutions:

- Replace tuna with canned salmon, grilled chicken, or hard-boiled eggs.
- Use chickpeas or black beans instead of white beans.
- Replace arugula with spinach, kale, or romaine lettuce.
- Add cucumber, bell peppers, or avocado for additional vegetables and healthy fats.
- Use red wine vinegar instead of lemon juice for a different flavor profile.
- Make it dairy-free by omitting feta cheese.

Storage & Meal Prep Tips: This salad can be made ahead and improves in flavor as it sits. Prepare the complete salad without greens and store in an airtight container in the refrigerator for up to 3 days. Add fresh greens just before serving to prevent wilting. The dressed bean and tuna mixture can marinate and develop flavor. This is an excellent make-ahead lunch option. Pack in containers with greens on the side, then combine when ready to eat.

Recipe 4: Asian-Inspired Beef and Broccoli Bowl

Prep Time: 10 minutes
Cook Time: 12 minutes
Servings: 2

Ingredients:

- 12 ounces flank steak or sirloin, thinly sliced against the grain
- 3 cups broccoli florets
- 1 red bell pepper, sliced
- 2 garlic cloves, minced
- 1 tablespoon fresh ginger, grated
- 3 tablespoons low-sodium soy sauce or coconut aminos
- 1 tablespoon rice vinegar

- 1 teaspoon sesame oil

- 1 tablespoon avocado oil or olive oil

- 1 teaspoon arrowroot powder or cornstarch

- ¼ teaspoon red pepper flakes (optional)

- 2 tablespoons sesame seeds

- 2 green onions, sliced

- Optional: 1 cup cooked brown rice or cauliflower rice per serving

Instructions:

1. In a small bowl, whisk together soy sauce, rice vinegar, sesame oil, arrowroot powder, and red pepper flakes if using. Set aside.

2. Heat avocado oil in a large skillet or wok over high heat.

3. Add sliced beef in a single layer. Cook without stirring for 2 minutes until browned on one side. Flip and cook for another 1 to 2 minutes. Remove beef from skillet and set aside.

4. In the same skillet, add broccoli florets and bell pepper. Stir-fry for 4 to 5 minutes until vegetables are tender-crisp. Add a splash of water if vegetables begin to stick.

5. Add minced garlic and grated ginger. Cook for 30 seconds until fragrant.

6. Return beef to the skillet.

7. Pour sauce over beef and vegetables. Toss to coat everything evenly. Cook for 1 to 2 minutes until sauce thickens slightly.

8. Remove from heat.

9. Divide between two bowls. If using, add cooked rice or cauliflower rice to each bowl.

10. Garnish with sesame seeds and sliced green onions.

Macronutrient Focus: High protein (approximately 38 grams), moderate fat (approximately 16 grams), low to moderate carbohydrate (approximately 14 grams without rice, 42 grams with brown rice). This is a protein-focused meal that can be adjusted for training needs.

Blood Sugar Impact: Minimal without rice, moderate with rice. The high protein from beef and fiber from vegetables create excellent blood sugar stability. Brown rice adds carbohydrates but remains balanced due to its fiber content and the high protein in the meal. This provides sustained energy without crashes.

Best Training-Day Pairing: Without rice, this is ideal for rest days or light activity days. With brown rice added, it becomes excellent for moderate to high training days, particularly after strength training. The protein supports muscle recovery. The iron and zinc from beef support overall health and hormone production.

Substitutions:

- Replace beef with chicken, shrimp, or tofu for different protein sources.

- Use snap peas, bok choy, or zucchini instead of broccoli.

- Replace brown rice with quinoa, white rice, or sweet potato for different carbohydrate sources.

- Use tamari instead of soy sauce for a gluten-free version.

- Add mushrooms, carrots, or water chestnuts for variety.

- Replace sesame oil with additional avocado oil if allergic to sesame.

Storage & Meal Prep Tips: This dish is excellent for meal prep but should be stored properly to maintain texture. Cook the beef and vegetable mixture and let cool completely. Store in airtight containers in the refrigerator for up to 4 days. Store rice separately. Reheat the beef and vegetables in a skillet or microwave, adding a splash of water to prevent drying. Reheat rice separately. For best texture, slightly undercook vegetables during initial prep, as they will soften further when reheated.

Recipe 5: Greek Lentil Soup

Prep Time: 10 minutes
Cook Time: 35 minutes
Servings: 4

Ingredients:

- 1½ cups dried green or brown lentils, rinsed

- 1 can (14.5 ounces) diced tomatoes

- 1 large onion, diced

- 2 carrots, diced

- 2 celery stalks, diced

- 3 garlic cloves, minced

- 6 cups low-sodium vegetable or chicken broth

- 2 tablespoons olive oil

- 2 tablespoons red wine vinegar

- 1 teaspoon dried oregano

- 1 teaspoon cumin

- 2 bay leaves

- Salt and black pepper to taste

- 2 cups fresh spinach or kale, chopped

- Optional: crumbled feta cheese and lemon wedges for serving

Instructions:

1. Heat olive oil in a large pot over medium heat.

2. Add diced onion, carrots, and celery. Sauté for 5 to 6 minutes until vegetables soften.

3. Add minced garlic, oregano, and cumin. Cook for 1 minute until fragrant.

4. Add rinsed lentils, diced tomatoes (with juice), broth, bay leaves, salt, and pepper.

5. Bring to a boil, then reduce heat to low and simmer, partially covered, for 25 to 30 minutes until lentils are tender.

6. Stir in red wine vinegar and chopped spinach or kale. Cook for 2 to 3 minutes until greens wilt.

7. Remove bay leaves.

8. Taste and adjust seasoning as needed.

9. Serve hot, topped with optional crumbled feta and a squeeze of lemon.

Macronutrient Focus: High protein (approximately 18 grams per serving), low fat (approximately 8 grams), moderate to high carbohydrate (approximately 42 grams). Lentils provide both protein and carbohydrates along with significant fiber.

Blood Sugar Impact: Low to moderate. Lentils are exceptionally high in fiber, which dramatically slows glucose absorption. Despite containing carbohydrates, lentils have one of the lowest glycemic impacts of any food. The combination of protein, fiber, and vegetables creates very stable blood sugar. This soup provides sustained energy for 4 to 5 hours.

Best Training-Day Pairing: Excellent for moderate to high training days. The carbohydrates from lentils provide fuel for strength training or cardio. This is ideal 2 to 3 hours before training or as a recovery meal. Also suitable for rest days due to the high fiber content, which prevents blood sugar spikes. The plant-based protein supports muscle maintenance.

Substitutions:

- Use red lentils for a creamier texture (reduce cooking time to 15 to 20 minutes as they cook faster).

- Add diced potatoes or sweet potatoes for additional carbohydrates on heavy training days.

- Replace spinach with Swiss chard or collard greens.

- Add a Parmesan rind during cooking for additional flavor (remove before serving).

- Make it heartier by adding diced cooked chicken or turkey sausage.

- Use fresh tomatoes instead of canned when in season.

Storage & Meal Prep Tips: This soup is ideal for meal prep and actually improves in flavor over time. Let cool completely and store in airtight containers in the refrigerator for up to 5 days or freeze for up to 3 months. The soup will thicken as it sits; add water or broth when reheating to reach desired consistency. Reheat on the stovetop or in the microwave. Freeze in individual portions for quick lunches. Add fresh greens and feta just before serving for best texture and flavor.

Recipe 6: Chicken and Quinoa Power Salad

Prep Time: 10 minutes
Cook Time: 20 minutes
Servings: 2

Ingredients:

- 12 ounces chicken breast

- 1 cup quinoa, uncooked

- 2 cups water or chicken broth

- 2 cups mixed greens or arugula

- 1 cup roasted sweet potato, cubed

- ½ cup dried cranberries or pomegranate seeds

- ¼ cup slivered almonds or pumpkin seeds

- ¼ cup crumbled goat cheese or feta

- 3 tablespoons olive oil

- 2 tablespoons balsamic vinegar

- 1 teaspoon Dijon mustard

- 1 teaspoon honey

- Salt and black pepper to taste

Instructions:

1. Cook quinoa: Rinse quinoa under cold water. In a medium pot, combine quinoa and water or broth. Bring to a boil, then reduce heat to low, cover, and simmer for 15 minutes until liquid is absorbed. Remove from heat and let sit covered for 5 minutes, then fluff with a fork.

2. While quinoa cooks, season chicken with salt and pepper. Grill, bake, or pan-sear chicken until cooked through (internal temperature of 165°F), about 6 to 8 minutes per side depending on thickness. Let rest for 5 minutes, then slice.

3. For the sweet potato, either roast cubed sweet potato at 425°F for 20 to 25 minutes until tender, or use leftover roasted sweet potato.

4. In a small bowl, whisk together olive oil, balsamic vinegar, Dijon mustard, honey, salt, and pepper to make the dressing.

5. Divide mixed greens between two large bowls.

6. Top each bowl with cooked quinoa, sliced chicken, roasted sweet potato, dried cranberries, almonds, and goat cheese.

7. Drizzle with balsamic dressing.

8. Toss before eating or eat in layers.

Macronutrient Focus: High protein (approximately 42 grams), moderate fat (approximately 20 grams), moderate to high carbohydrate (approximately 58 grams). This is a balanced, nutrient-dense meal with carbohydrates from quinoa and sweet potato.

Blood Sugar Impact: Low to moderate. Quinoa and sweet potato both have relatively low glycemic indices, especially when combined with the high protein from chicken and healthy fats from olive oil and nuts. The fiber from vegetables, quinoa, and sweet potato further stabilizes blood sugar. This meal provides sustained energy for 4 to 5 hours.

Best Training-Day Pairing: Excellent for moderate to high training days, particularly after strength training or as a pre-training meal 2 to 3 hours before exercise. The carbohydrates support glycogen replenishment and provide energy. The protein supports muscle recovery. This is also suitable after long Zone 2 cardio sessions. For rest days, reduce quinoa and sweet potato portions.

Substitutions:

- Replace chicken with salmon, shrimp, or chickpeas for a vegetarian version.

- Use brown rice, farro, or couscous instead of quinoa.

- Replace sweet potato with butternut squash, roasted beets, or additional vegetables.

- Use pecans, walnuts, or sunflower seeds instead of almonds.

- Replace dried cranberries with fresh berries, apple slices, or raisins.

- Use blue cheese or omit cheese for dairy-free.

- Replace balsamic dressing with lemon vinaigrette or tahini dressing.

Storage & Meal Prep Tips: This salad is excellent for meal prep. Cook quinoa, chicken, and sweet potato in bulk at the beginning of the week. Store each component separately in airtight containers in the refrigerator for up to 4 days. Wash and store greens separately. Store dressing in a small jar or container. Assemble salads each day or assemble complete salads without dressing and store for up to 3 days. Add dressing just before eating. This prevents wilting and maintains texture.

Recipe 7: Egg Salad Lettuce Wraps

Prep Time: 15 minutes
Cook Time: 0 minutes (assuming eggs are pre-cooked)
Servings: 2

Ingredients:

- 6 hard-boiled eggs, peeled and chopped

- 3 tablespoons Greek yogurt or mayonnaise

- 1 teaspoon Dijon mustard

- 2 celery stalks, finely diced

- 2 tablespoons fresh chives or green onions, chopped

- 1 teaspoon fresh dill, chopped (or ½ teaspoon dried)

- Salt and black pepper to taste

- 8 large lettuce leaves (butter lettuce, romaine, or iceberg)

- 1 avocado, sliced

- 1 cup cherry tomatoes, halved

- Optional: everything bagel seasoning

Instructions:

1. In a medium bowl, combine chopped hard-boiled eggs, Greek yogurt or mayonnaise, and Dijon mustard. Mix well.

2. Add diced celery, chives or green onions, and dill. Stir to combine.

3. Season with salt and black pepper to taste.

4. Wash and dry lettuce leaves. Pat completely dry.

5. Divide egg salad among lettuce leaves, placing a generous spoonful in the center of each.

6. Top with avocado slices and cherry tomatoes.

7. Sprinkle with optional everything bagel seasoning.

8. Fold lettuce leaves like tacos or wraps and eat with your hands.

Macronutrient Focus: High protein (approximately 24 grams per serving), high fat (approximately 28 grams), very low carbohydrate (approximately 8 grams). This is a protein and fat-focused meal ideal for low-carb days.

Blood Sugar Impact: Minimal to none. Eggs provide protein and fat with virtually no carbohydrates. The small amount of carbohydrates from vegetables has negligible impact. This meal produces extremely stable blood sugar and sustained satiety.

Best Training-Day Pairing: Ideal for rest days or light activity days due to very low carbohydrate content. Also excellent for post-Zone 2 cardio when carbohydrate needs are minimal. For moderate to high training days, pair with fruit, sweet potato, or whole grain crackers to increase carbohydrates.

Substitutions:

- Replace hard-boiled eggs with canned tuna or chicken for variety.

- Use all mayonnaise or all Greek yogurt based on preference (Greek yogurt reduces fat and increases protein).

- Add diced pickles, capers, or jalapeños for additional flavor.

- Use cabbage leaves or collard greens instead of lettuce for sturdier wraps.

- Replace avocado with hummus or roasted red peppers.

- Add sprouts, cucumber, or shredded carrots for additional crunch.

Storage & Meal Prep Tips: Hard-boil eggs at the beginning of the week and store unpeeled in the refrigerator for up to 5 days. Prepare egg salad up to 3 days in advance and store in an airtight container in the refrigerator. Assemble wraps fresh each day for best texture. If packing for lunch, store egg salad in one container and lettuce leaves in another, then assemble just before eating. This prevents lettuce from becoming soggy. Wash and dry lettuce in advance and store wrapped in paper towels in a container or plastic bag.

Recipe 8: Hearty Vegetable and Chicken Stew

Prep Time: 15 minutes
Cook Time: 35 minutes
Servings: 4

Ingredients:

- 1 pound boneless, skinless chicken thighs, cut into bite-sized pieces

- 2 tablespoons olive oil

- 1 large onion, diced

- 3 garlic cloves, minced

- 3 carrots, peeled and sliced

- 2 celery stalks, sliced

- 2 medium zucchini, diced

- 1 can (14.5 ounces) diced tomatoes

- 4 cups low-sodium chicken broth

- 1 can (15 ounces) white beans, drained and rinsed

- 2 cups fresh spinach or kale, chopped

- 1 teaspoon dried thyme

- 1 teaspoon dried rosemary

- 1 bay leaf

- Salt and black pepper to taste

- Optional: grated Parmesan cheese for serving

Instructions:

1. Heat 1 tablespoon of olive oil in a large pot over medium-high heat.

2. Season chicken pieces with salt and pepper. Add to pot and cook for 5 to 6 minutes until browned on all sides. Remove chicken and set aside.

3. Add remaining 1 tablespoon of olive oil to the pot. Add diced onion, carrots, and celery. Sauté for 5 to 6 minutes until vegetables begin to soften.

4. Add minced garlic, thyme, and rosemary. Cook for 1 minute until fragrant.

5. Add chicken broth, diced tomatoes (with juice), bay leaf, and browned chicken pieces. Bring to a boil.

6. Reduce heat to low and simmer, partially covered, for 15 minutes.

7. Add diced zucchini and white beans. Simmer for another 10 minutes until all vegetables are tender.

8. Stir in chopped spinach or kale. Cook for 2 to 3 minutes until wilted.

9. Remove bay leaf.

10. Taste and adjust seasoning as needed.

11. Serve hot, topped with optional grated Parmesan cheese.

Macronutrient Focus: High protein (approximately 32 grams per serving), low fat (approximately 10 grams), moderate carbohydrate (approximately 28 grams). This is a lean, nutrient-dense meal with protein from chicken and beans.

Blood Sugar Impact: Low to moderate. White beans provide fiber that slows glucose absorption. The high protein from chicken and beans, combined with fiber from vegetables, creates very stable blood sugar. This stew provides sustained energy and satiety for 4 to 5 hours.

Best Training-Day Pairing: Suitable for moderate training days or as a recovery meal after strength training or Zone 2 cardio. The carbohydrates from beans support glycogen replenishment without being excessive. Also excellent for rest days due to balanced macronutrients. The lean protein supports muscle recovery and maintenance.

Substitutions:

- Replace chicken thighs with chicken breast for leaner protein (though thighs are more flavorful and stay moist).

- Use turkey, ground turkey, or omit meat entirely for a vegetarian version.

- Replace white beans with chickpeas, kidney beans, or lentils.

- Add potatoes or sweet potatoes for additional carbohydrates on heavy training days.

- Use Swiss chard, collard greens, or cabbage instead of spinach.

- Add mushrooms, bell peppers, or green beans for variety.

Storage & Meal Prep Tips: This stew is ideal for meal prep and freezes beautifully. Let cool completely and store in airtight containers in the refrigerator for up to 5 days or freeze for up to 3 months. The stew will thicken as it sits; add water or broth when reheating to reach desired consistency. Reheat on the stovetop or in the microwave. Freeze in individual portions for easy grab-and-go lunches. Add fresh greens and Parmesan just before serving for best flavor and texture.

Recipe 9: Shrimp and Avocado Salad

Prep Time: 10 minutes
Cook Time: 5 minutes
Servings: 2

Ingredients:

- 12 ounces raw shrimp, peeled and deveined

- 4 cups mixed greens or butter lettuce

- 1 avocado, diced

- 1 cup cherry tomatoes, halved

- 1 cucumber, sliced

- ¼ cup red onion, thinly sliced

- ¼ cup fresh cilantro, chopped

- 3 tablespoons olive oil

- 2 tablespoons lime juice

- 1 garlic clove, minced

- ½ teaspoon cumin

- ½ teaspoon chili powder

- Salt and black pepper to taste

- Optional: crumbled queso fresco or feta cheese

Instructions:

1. Pat shrimp dry with paper towels. Season with cumin, chili powder, salt, and pepper.

2. Heat 1 tablespoon of olive oil in a skillet over medium-high heat.

3. Add shrimp in a single layer. Cook for 2 minutes per side until pink and opaque. Remove from heat.

4. In a small bowl, whisk together remaining 2 tablespoons of olive oil, lime juice, minced garlic, salt, and pepper to make the dressing.

5. Divide mixed greens between two bowls or plates.

6. Top each bowl with cooked shrimp, diced avocado, cherry tomatoes, cucumber, red onion, and fresh cilantro.

7. Drizzle with lime dressing.

8. Top with optional crumbled cheese.

9. Toss before eating or eat in layers.

Macronutrient Focus: High protein (approximately 36 grams), moderate fat (approximately 24 grams), low carbohydrate (approximately 16 grams). This is a protein and healthy fat-focused meal.

Blood Sugar Impact: Minimal. Shrimp provides lean protein with virtually no carbohydrates. Avocado adds healthy fats. Vegetables provide fiber. This meal has minimal impact on blood sugar and provides sustained satiety.

Best Training-Day Pairing: Ideal for rest days or light activity days due to low carbohydrate content. Also excellent after Zone 2 cardio when carbohydrate needs are moderate. For heavy training days, pair with quinoa, brown rice, or sweet potato to increase carbohydrates. The lean protein from shrimp supports muscle recovery without excess calories.

Substitutions:

- Replace shrimp with grilled chicken, salmon, or scallops.

- Use romaine lettuce, arugula, or spinach instead of mixed greens.

- Add corn, black beans, or bell peppers for additional vegetables and carbohydrates.

- Replace cilantro with fresh basil or parsley if you dislike cilantro.

- Use lemon juice instead of lime juice for a different flavor.

- Make it dairy-free by omitting cheese.

Storage & Meal Prep Tips: This salad is best assembled fresh, but components can be prepped in advance. Cook shrimp up to 2 days ahead and store in the refrigerator. Wash and chop vegetables and store in separate containers. Store dressing separately. Assemble salads each day for best texture. If you must assemble ahead, keep avocado and dressing separate until ready to eat to prevent browning and wilting. Squeeze lime juice over avocado to prevent oxidation if preparing in advance.

Recipe 10: Turkey Meatball and Zucchini Noodle Bowl

Prep Time: 15 minutes
Cook Time: 20 minutes
Servings: 2

Ingredients:

For Meatballs:

- 1 pound ground turkey (93% lean)

- 1 egg

- ¼ cup almond flour or breadcrumbs

- 2 garlic cloves, minced

- 1 teaspoon Italian seasoning

- ½ teaspoon salt

- ¼ teaspoon black pepper

- 2 tablespoons grated Parmesan cheese

For Bowl:

- 3 medium zucchini, spiralized into noodles

- 2 cups marinara sauce (look for low-sugar versions)

- 1 tablespoon olive oil

- Fresh basil for garnish

- Optional: additional grated Parmesan cheese

Instructions:

1. Preheat oven to 400°F (200°C). Line a baking sheet with parchment paper.

2. In a large bowl, combine ground turkey, egg, almond flour, minced garlic, Italian seasoning, salt, pepper, and Parmesan cheese. Mix gently until just combined (do not overmix).

3. Form mixture into 12 to 14 meatballs, about 1.5 inches in diameter.

4. Place meatballs on the prepared baking sheet. Bake for 18 to 20 minutes until cooked through (internal temperature of 165°F) and lightly browned.

5. While meatballs bake, heat marinara sauce in a medium pot over low heat.

6. Heat olive oil in a large skillet over medium heat. Add spiralized zucchini noodles and sauté for 2 to 3 minutes until just tender (do not overcook or they will become watery). Season with salt and pepper.

7. Divide zucchini noodles between two bowls.

8. Top each bowl with warm marinara sauce and cooked meatballs.

9. Garnish with fresh basil and optional Parmesan cheese.

Macronutrient Focus: High protein (approximately 42 grams), moderate fat (approximately 18 grams), low carbohydrate (approximately 20 grams). This is a high-protein, lower-carbohydrate alternative to traditional pasta.

Blood Sugar Impact: Low. Zucchini noodles are very low in carbohydrates compared to pasta. The marinara sauce contains some carbohydrates from tomatoes, but the high protein from turkey meatballs creates excellent blood sugar stability. This meal provides sustained energy without spikes or crashes.

Best Training-Day Pairing: Suitable for rest days or light activity days due to lower carbohydrate content. For moderate to high training days, add whole grain pasta alongside or instead of zucchini noodles to increase carbohydrates. Also excellent for post-workout when you want protein without excessive carbohydrates.

Substitutions:

- Replace ground turkey with ground chicken, beef, or plant-based meat alternative.

- Use regular pasta, whole wheat pasta, or spaghetti squash instead of zucchini noodles for different carbohydrate levels.

- Replace almond flour with regular breadcrumbs or oat flour.

- Make meatballs dairy-free by omitting Parmesan (they will be slightly less moist).

- Add vegetables to the marinara sauce: mushrooms, bell peppers, or spinach.

- Use pesto or Alfredo sauce instead of marinara for variety.

Storage & Meal Prep Tips: Meatballs are excellent for meal prep. Cook meatballs and let cool completely. Store in an airtight container in the refrigerator for up to 4 days or freeze for up to 3 months. Reheat in marinara sauce on the stovetop or in the microwave. Zucchini noodles are best made fresh, as they become watery when stored. However, you can spiralize zucchini in advance and store raw noodles in a container lined with paper towels for up to 2 days. Sauté just before serving. Store marinara sauce separately.

Recipe 11: Salmon and Roasted Vegetable Plate

Prep Time: 10 minutes
Cook Time: 20 minutes
Servings: 2

Ingredients:

- 2 salmon fillets (5-6 ounces each)

- 2 cups Brussels sprouts, halved

- 1 cup cherry tomatoes

- 1 red bell pepper, cut into chunks

- 1 red onion, cut into wedges

- 3 tablespoons olive oil, divided

- 2 garlic cloves, minced

- 1 lemon, sliced

- 1 teaspoon dried dill or fresh dill

- Salt and black pepper to taste

- Optional: 2 tablespoons balsamic glaze for drizzling

Instructions:

1. Preheat oven to 425°F (220°C). Line a large baking sheet with parchment paper.

2. Place Brussels sprouts, cherry tomatoes, bell pepper, and red onion on the baking sheet. Drizzle with 2 tablespoons of olive oil, season with salt and pepper, and toss to coat. Spread vegetables in a single layer.

3. Roast vegetables for 10 minutes.

4. While vegetables roast, pat salmon fillets dry with paper towels. Rub with remaining 1 tablespoon of olive oil and minced garlic. Season with dill, salt, and pepper.

5. After 10 minutes, remove baking sheet from oven. Push vegetables to the sides and place salmon fillets in the center. Top each fillet with lemon slices.

6. Return to oven and roast for 10 to 12 minutes until salmon flakes easily with a fork and vegetables are caramelized.

7. Divide vegetables and salmon between two plates.

8. Drizzle with optional balsamic glaze.

Macronutrient Focus: High protein (approximately 35 grams), moderate fat (approximately 22 grams, mostly omega-3s), low to moderate carbohydrate (approximately 18 grams). This is a nutrient-dense meal rich in anti-inflammatory omega-3 fatty acids.

Blood Sugar Impact: Low. Salmon provides protein and healthy fats with no carbohydrates. Vegetables provide fiber and minimal carbohydrates. This meal has very low glycemic impact and provides stable, sustained energy.

Best Training-Day Pairing: Suitable for rest days or light activity days. The omega-3s from salmon support recovery and reduce inflammation, making this excellent any time. For moderate to high training days, add quinoa, brown rice, or sweet potato to increase carbohydrates. Also ideal after Zone 2 cardio or strength training when you want protein and anti-inflammatory fats without excess carbohydrates.

Substitutions:

- Replace salmon with cod, halibut, or chicken breast.

- Use any combination of vegetables: broccoli, asparagus, zucchini, cauliflower, or sweet potato.

- Replace fresh dill with other herbs: thyme, rosemary, or parsley.

- Add capers or olives for additional flavor.

- Use lime instead of lemon for a different citrus profile.

Storage & Meal Prep Tips: This meal can be partially prepped in advance. Chop vegetables and store in containers for up to 3 days. Roast salmon and vegetables together and store in airtight containers in the refrigerator for up to 3 days. Reheat gently in a 350°F oven for 10 minutes or in the microwave. Salmon is best fresh but reheats reasonably well. You can also cook extra salmon and serve it cold on salads for variety throughout the week.

Recipe 12: Chicken Caesar Salad (Longevity Version)

Prep Time: 10 minutes
Cook Time: 10 minutes
Servings: 2

Ingredients:

For Salad:

- 12 ounces chicken breast

- 4 cups romaine lettuce, chopped

- ¼ cup grated Parmesan cheese

- Optional: 1 cup whole grain croutons or chickpea croutons

For Dressing:

- ¼ cup Greek yogurt

- 2 tablespoons olive oil

- 2 tablespoons lemon juice

- 2 garlic cloves, minced

- 2 teaspoons Dijon mustard

- 2 teaspoons Worcestershire sauce

- ¼ cup grated Parmesan cheese

- Salt and black pepper to taste

- Water to thin if needed

Instructions:

1. Season chicken breast with salt and pepper. Grill, bake, or pan-sear until cooked through (internal temperature of 165°F), about 6 to 8 minutes per side. Let rest for 5 minutes, then slice.

2. While chicken cooks, prepare dressing: In a small bowl or jar, combine Greek yogurt, olive oil, lemon juice, minced garlic, Dijon mustard, Worcestershire sauce, Parmesan cheese, salt, and pepper. Whisk or shake until smooth. Add water 1 tablespoon at a time if dressing is too thick.

3. Place chopped romaine lettuce in a large bowl.

4. Add sliced chicken, grated Parmesan cheese, and optional croutons.

5. Drizzle with Caesar dressing and toss to coat.

6. Divide between two plates and serve immediately.

Macronutrient Focus: High protein (approximately 40 grams without croutons, 44 grams with), moderate fat (approximately 16 grams), low carbohydrate (approximately 8 grams without croutons, 24 grams with). This version uses Greek yogurt to reduce fat while maintaining creaminess and increasing protein.

Blood Sugar Impact: Minimal without croutons, low to moderate with croutons. The high protein from chicken and Greek yogurt creates excellent satiety and blood sugar stability. Whole grain croutons add some carbohydrates but remain balanced due to fiber and protein content.

Best Training-Day Pairing: Without croutons, ideal for rest days or light activity days. With croutons, suitable for moderate training days or post-Zone 2 cardio. For heavy training days, add additional croutons or serve with whole grain bread. The lean protein supports muscle recovery and maintenance.

Substitutions:

- Replace chicken with grilled shrimp, salmon, or hard-boiled eggs.

- Use kale instead of romaine for additional nutrients (massage kale with a bit of dressing to soften).

- Make croutons from whole grain bread: cube bread, toss with olive oil and garlic, and bake at 375°F for 10 minutes.

- Use roasted chickpeas instead of croutons for additional protein and fiber.

- Make it dairy-free by omitting Parmesan and using nutritional yeast for savory flavor.

- Add anchovies to the dressing for traditional Caesar flavor (optional).

Storage & Meal Prep Tips: Cook chicken in bulk and store in the refrigerator for up to 4 days. Make dressing up to 5 days in advance and store in an airtight jar or container in the refrigerator. Wash and chop lettuce and store wrapped in paper towels in an airtight container for up to 3 days. Assemble salads fresh each day for best texture, or pack components separately and combine just before eating. Never dress salad in advance, as lettuce will wilt. Keep dressing separate until ready to eat.

These twelve lunch recipes provide substantial variety while maintaining the core principles of longevity nutrition. Each recipe prioritizes protein for muscle maintenance and satiety, includes vegetables for fiber and micronutrients, and offers flexibility with carbohydrate content based on training demands.

Several recipes are ideal for meal prep, allowing you to cook once and eat multiple times throughout the week. Others come together quickly for days when you have time to prepare fresh meals. Many are portable, making them suitable for taking to work or eating on the go.

As with breakfast, these recipes are templates. Adjust portions based on your body size, activity level, and training schedule. Swap ingredients based on preferences and availability. The principles remain constant: build meals around protein, include plenty of vegetables, choose quality carbohydrates when needed, and incorporate healthy fats.

Pay attention to how these meals make you feel. Do they keep you satisfied until dinner? Do you have stable energy throughout the afternoon? Are you recovering well from training? Use this feedback to adjust portions and macronutrient ratios.

Lunch is not a break from your nutrition plan. It is an opportunity to fuel your body for the rest of the day, support your training, and move closer to your longevity goals. Make it count.

Dinner is the meal where most people finally have time to slow down, cook, and eat mindfully. After a day of work, training, and navigating countless decisions, dinner becomes an anchor, a ritual that signals the transition from doing to recovering.

Yet dinner is also where discipline often breaks down. You arrive home tired and hungry. The temptation to order takeout, eat whatever is easiest, or mindlessly snack while cooking is strong. Without a plan, dinner defaults to convenience rather than intention.

A well-constructed dinner should accomplish several things. It should provide adequate protein to support overnight muscle repair and recovery. It should include vegetables for fiber, micronutrients, and satiety. It should contain appropriate carbohydrates based on your training schedule and activity level. And critically, it should be satisfying enough to prevent late-night snacking driven by inadequate nutrition.

This chapter provides eighteen dinner recipes that meet these criteria. They range from quick thirty-minute meals for busy weeknights to slower-cooked comfort foods that can simmer while you handle other tasks. Each recipe includes detailed preparation guidance, macronutrient information, blood sugar impact, training-day pairing recommendations, substitutions, and meal prep strategies.

These are real dinners for real people. They taste good. They satisfy. They support your goals without requiring perfection or sacrifice. And most importantly, they are recipes you will actually make and eat consistently.

Let's begin.

Recipe 1: Herb-Roasted Chicken with Root Vegetables

Prep Time: 15 minutes
Cook Time: 45 minutes
Servings: 4

Ingredients:

- 4 bone-in, skin-on chicken thighs

- 3 large carrots, peeled and cut into chunks

- 2 parsnips, peeled and cut into chunks

- 1 pound baby potatoes, halved

- 1 large red onion, cut into wedges

- 4 garlic cloves, smashed

- 3 tablespoons olive oil

- 2 tablespoons fresh rosemary, chopped (or 2 teaspoons dried)

- 1 tablespoon fresh thyme, chopped (or 1 teaspoon dried)

- 1 teaspoon paprika

- Salt and black pepper to taste

- 1 lemon, cut into wedges

Instructions:

1. Preheat oven to 425°F (220°C).

2. In a large bowl, toss carrots, parsnips, potatoes, red onion, and smashed garlic with 2 tablespoons of olive oil. Season with half the rosemary, half the thyme, salt, and pepper. Spread vegetables in a single layer on a large baking sheet or roasting pan.

3. Pat chicken thighs dry with paper towels. Rub with remaining 1 tablespoon of olive oil. Season both sides generously with remaining rosemary, thyme, paprika, salt, and pepper.

4. Place chicken thighs on top of the vegetables, skin side up.

5. Roast for 40 to 45 minutes until chicken skin is crispy and golden and internal temperature reaches 165°F. Vegetables should be tender and caramelized.

6. Remove from oven and let rest for 5 minutes.

7. Squeeze fresh lemon juice over chicken and vegetables before serving.

8. Divide chicken and vegetables among four plates.

Macronutrient Focus: High protein (approximately 32 grams), moderate fat (approximately 18 grams), moderate carbohydrate (approximately 35 grams). This is a balanced, complete meal with protein from chicken and carbohydrates from root vegetables.

Blood Sugar Impact: Low to moderate. Root vegetables have moderate carbohydrate content, but their fiber slows glucose absorption. The high protein and fat from chicken thighs creates excellent satiety and stable blood sugar. This meal provides sustained energy and fullness for 4 to 5 hours.

Best Training-Day Pairing: Excellent for moderate to high training days, particularly after strength training or intense cardio. The carbohydrates from potatoes and root vegetables support glycogen replenishment. The protein supports muscle recovery. Also suitable for rest days if you reduce the potato portion or substitute with additional non-starchy vegetables.

Substitutions:

- Replace chicken thighs with chicken breast (reduce cooking time to 30 to 35 minutes).

- Use sweet potatoes instead of regular potatoes for different nutrients.

- Replace parsnips with turnips, rutabaga, or additional carrots.

- Add Brussels sprouts, bell peppers, or fennel for variety.

- Use bone-in pork chops instead of chicken for a different protein.

- Make it lower-carb by replacing potatoes with cauliflower florets.

Storage & Meal Prep Tips: This is an excellent sheet-pan meal for meal prep. Let chicken and vegetables cool completely, then divide into airtight containers. Store in the refrigerator for up to 4 days. Reheat in a 350°F oven for 15 minutes or in the microwave. The chicken skin will lose some crispness when reheated but remains flavorful. For best results, reheat in the oven. You can also shred the chicken after cooking and use it in salads, wraps, or bowls throughout the week.

Recipe 2: Grilled Steak with Chimichurri and Roasted Broccoli

Prep Time: 15 minutes
Cook Time: 20 minutes
Servings: 2

Ingredients:

For Steak:

- 2 sirloin or ribeye steaks (6-8 ounces each)

- 2 tablespoons olive oil

- Salt and black pepper to taste

For Chimichurri:

- 1 cup fresh parsley, finely chopped

- ¼ cup fresh cilantro, finely chopped

- 3 garlic cloves, minced

- 2 tablespoons red wine vinegar

- ½ cup olive oil

- ½ teaspoon red pepper flakes

- Salt and black pepper to taste

For Broccoli:

- 4 cups broccoli florets

- 2 tablespoons olive oil

- 2 garlic cloves, minced

- Salt, black pepper, and lemon zest to taste

Instructions:

1. Preheat oven to 425°F (220°C) for the broccoli. If grilling steak, preheat grill to high heat. If pan-searing, wait until broccoli goes in the oven.

2. Make chimichurri: In a medium bowl, combine chopped parsley, cilantro, minced garlic, red wine vinegar, olive oil, red pepper flakes, salt, and pepper. Mix well and set aside to let flavors meld.

3. Prepare broccoli: Toss broccoli florets with olive oil, minced garlic, salt, and pepper. Spread in a single layer on a baking sheet. Roast for 18 to 20 minutes until tender and edges are crispy and caramelized. Finish with lemon zest.

4. While broccoli roasts, prepare steak: Pat steaks dry with paper towels. Rub both sides with olive oil and season generously with salt and pepper. Let sit at room temperature for 10 minutes.

5. For grilling: Place steaks on hot grill. Cook for 4 to 5 minutes per side for medium-rare (internal temperature of 130-135°F), or adjust time based on desired doneness. For pan-searing: Heat a cast iron skillet over high heat until smoking. Add steaks and cook for 4 to 5 minutes per side.

6. Remove steaks from heat and let rest for 5 to 10 minutes before slicing.

7. Slice steak against the grain.

8. Divide steak and roasted broccoli between two plates.

9. Top steak generously with chimichurri sauce.

Macronutrient Focus: High protein (approximately 42 grams), high fat (approximately 38 grams), low carbohydrate (approximately 12 grams). This is a protein and fat-focused meal with minimal carbohydrates.

Blood Sugar Impact: Minimal. Steak provides protein and fat with no carbohydrates. Broccoli provides fiber and minimal carbohydrates. This meal has virtually no impact on blood sugar and provides excellent satiety.

Best Training-Day Pairing: Ideal for rest days or light activity days due to low carbohydrate content. The high protein and iron from steak support recovery and hormone health. For moderate to high training days, add roasted potatoes, sweet potato, or quinoa to increase carbohydrates. The chimichurri provides anti-inflammatory herbs and healthy fats.

Substitutions:

- Replace sirloin with flank steak, skirt steak, or tenderloin.

- Use grilled chicken, pork chops, or salmon instead of beef.

- Replace broccoli with asparagus, green beans, or Brussels sprouts.

- Make chimichurri with all parsley if you dislike cilantro.

- Add roasted bell peppers or zucchini for additional vegetables.

Storage & Meal Prep Tips: Chimichurri can be made up to 5 days in advance and stored in an airtight jar in the refrigerator. The flavors actually improve over time. Cooked steak can be stored in the refrigerator for up to 3 days, but it is best enjoyed fresh. Slice leftover steak and use in salads, wraps, or grain bowls. Roasted broccoli can be prepped and reheated, though it loses some texture. Store in an airtight container for up to 4 days. For meal prep, cook components separately and assemble fresh meals throughout the week.

Recipe 3: Baked Salmon with Lemon-Dill Sauce and Asparagus

Prep Time: 10 minutes
Cook Time: 15 minutes
Servings: 2

Ingredients:

For Salmon:

- 2 salmon fillets (5-6 ounces each)
- 1 tablespoon olive oil
- 1 teaspoon garlic powder
- Salt and black pepper to taste
- 1 lemon, sliced

For Asparagus:

- 1 pound asparagus, tough ends trimmed
- 1 tablespoon olive oil
- Salt and black pepper to taste

For Lemon-Dill Sauce:

- ¼ cup Greek yogurt
- 1 tablespoon fresh dill, chopped (or 1 teaspoon dried)
- 1 tablespoon lemon juice
- 1 teaspoon lemon zest
- 1 garlic clove, minced
- Salt and black pepper to taste

Instructions:

1. Preheat oven to 400°F (200°C). Line a baking sheet with parchment paper.

2. Place asparagus on one side of the baking sheet. Drizzle with olive oil and season with salt and pepper. Toss to coat.

3. Pat salmon fillets dry with paper towels. Rub with olive oil and season with garlic powder, salt, and pepper. Place salmon on the other side of the baking sheet. Top each fillet with lemon slices.

4. Bake for 12 to 15 minutes until salmon flakes easily with a fork and asparagus is tender and slightly caramelized.

5. While salmon and asparagus bake, make the sauce: In a small bowl, combine Greek yogurt, fresh dill, lemon juice, lemon zest, minced garlic, salt, and pepper. Mix well.

6. Remove salmon and asparagus from oven.

7. Divide between two plates and drizzle salmon with lemon-dill sauce.

Macronutrient Focus: High protein (approximately 36 grams), moderate fat (approximately 20 grams, mostly omega-3s), low carbohydrate (approximately 8 grams). This is a lean, nutrient-dense meal rich in anti-inflammatory fats.

Blood Sugar Impact: Minimal. Salmon provides protein and omega-3 fatty acids with no carbohydrates. Asparagus provides fiber and minimal carbohydrates. This meal has negligible impact on blood sugar.

Best Training-Day Pairing: Suitable for rest days or light activity days. The omega-3s from salmon reduce inflammation and support recovery, making this excellent after any training. For moderate to high training days, add quinoa, brown rice, or roasted potatoes to increase carbohydrates. Also ideal after Zone 2 cardio or strength training when you want protein without excess carbohydrates.

Substitutions:

- Replace salmon with cod, halibut, trout, or chicken breast.

- Use green beans, broccoli, or Brussels sprouts instead of asparagus.

- Replace Greek yogurt sauce with hollandaise, pesto, or simply butter and lemon.

- Add capers to the sauce for additional flavor.

- Use fresh basil or parsley instead of dill.

Storage & Meal Prep Tips: Salmon is best fresh but can be stored in the refrigerator for up to 2 days. Reheat gently to avoid drying out, or serve cold on salads. Asparagus can be roasted ahead and stored for up to 3 days, though texture will soften. Make the lemon-dill sauce up to 3 days in advance and store in an airtight container. For meal prep, cook extra salmon and vegetables to use in various meals throughout the week. Cold salmon is excellent on salads or in wraps.

Recipe 4: Turkey and Vegetable Stuffed Peppers

Prep Time: 15 minutes
Cook Time: 40 minutes
Servings: 4

Ingredients:

- 4 large bell peppers (any color), tops cut off and seeds removed

- 1 pound ground turkey (93% lean)

- 1 cup cooked brown rice or cauliflower rice

- 1 can (14.5 ounces) diced tomatoes, drained

- 1 small zucchini, diced

- ½ cup onion, diced

- 2 garlic cloves, minced

- 1 cup shredded mozzarella or Mexican blend cheese, divided

- 1 teaspoon Italian seasoning

- 1 teaspoon cumin

- Salt and black pepper to taste

- 2 tablespoons olive oil

- Optional: fresh basil or cilantro for garnish

Instructions:

1. Preheat oven to 375°F (190°C).

2. Place bell peppers upright in a baking dish. If they don't stand upright, slice a small amount off the bottom to create a flat base (being careful not to create a hole).

3. Heat olive oil in a large skillet over medium heat. Add diced onion and cook for 3 to 4 minutes until softened.

4. Add ground turkey to the skillet, breaking it up with a spatula. Cook for 6 to 8 minutes until browned and cooked through.

5. Add minced garlic, diced zucchini, Italian seasoning, cumin, salt, and pepper. Cook for 3 to 4 minutes until zucchini softens.

6. Stir in cooked rice, diced tomatoes, and half the shredded cheese. Mix until combined and heated through.

7. Spoon the turkey mixture into each bell pepper, packing firmly. Top each pepper with remaining cheese.

8. Cover the baking dish with foil and bake for 25 minutes.

9. Remove foil and bake for an additional 10 to 15 minutes until peppers are tender and cheese is melted and bubbly.

10. Remove from oven and let cool for 5 minutes.

11. Garnish with fresh basil or cilantro if using.

Macronutrient Focus: High protein (approximately 28 grams per serving), moderate fat (approximately 12 grams), moderate carbohydrate (approximately 24 grams with brown rice, 10 grams with cauliflower rice). This is a balanced, veggie-forward meal.

Blood Sugar Impact: Low to moderate with brown rice, minimal with cauliflower rice. Bell peppers provide fiber and vitamins with minimal impact on blood sugar. Brown rice adds carbohydrates but remains balanced due to fiber and high protein content. Cauliflower rice version has negligible blood sugar impact.

Best Training-Day Pairing: With brown rice, excellent for moderate training days or post-strength training. With cauliflower rice, ideal for rest days or light activity days. The lean protein from turkey supports muscle recovery. This is a complete, satisfying meal that works for various training schedules.

Substitutions:

- Replace ground turkey with ground chicken, beef, or plant-based meat alternative.

- Use quinoa, wild rice, or farro instead of brown rice.

- Add black beans or lentils for additional protein and fiber.

- Use diced tomatoes with green chilies for a spicier version.

- Replace mozzarella with cheddar, pepper jack, or omit cheese for dairy-free.

- Add corn, mushrooms, or spinach to the filling for additional vegetables.

Storage & Meal Prep Tips: Stuffed peppers are ideal for meal prep. Let cool completely and store in airtight containers in the refrigerator for up to 4 days or freeze for up to 3 months. Reheat in a 350°F oven for 20 minutes or in the microwave. The peppers actually taste better the next day as flavors meld. You can also prepare the filling in advance, stuff the peppers, and refrigerate uncooked for up to 24 hours before baking. For freezing, wrap individual peppers in foil, then place in freezer bags. Thaw overnight in the refrigerator before reheating.

Recipe 5: One-Pan Lemon Garlic Chicken and Green Beans

Prep Time: 10 minutes
Cook Time: 25 minutes
Servings: 2

Ingredients:

- 2 boneless, skinless chicken breasts (6 ounces each)
- 1 pound green beans, trimmed
- 3 tablespoons olive oil, divided
- 4 garlic cloves, minced
- 1 lemon, zested and juiced
- 1 teaspoon dried oregano
- ½ teaspoon paprika
- Salt and black pepper to taste
- Optional: red pepper flakes for heat

Instructions:

1. Preheat oven to 400°F (200°C).
2. Pat chicken breasts dry with paper towels. Season both sides with oregano, paprika, salt, and pepper.
3. Heat 1 tablespoon of olive oil in a large oven-safe skillet over medium-high heat.
4. Add chicken breasts and sear for 3 to 4 minutes per side until golden brown. Remove chicken from skillet and set aside.
5. In the same skillet, add remaining 2 tablespoons of olive oil. Add green beans and minced garlic. Sauté for 2 to 3 minutes until fragrant.
6. Add lemon zest, lemon juice, salt, pepper, and optional red pepper flakes. Toss to coat green beans.
7. Nestle the seared chicken breasts into the green beans.
8. Transfer the skillet to the oven and bake for 12 to 15 minutes until chicken reaches an internal temperature of 165°F and green beans are tender.
9. Remove from oven and let rest for 5 minutes.
10. Divide chicken and green beans between two plates. Drizzle with any remaining pan juices.

Macronutrient Focus: High protein (approximately 42 grams), moderate fat (approximately 18 grams), low carbohydrate (approximately 12 grams). This is a lean, simple meal focused on protein and vegetables.

Blood Sugar Impact: Minimal. Chicken provides lean protein with no carbohydrates. Green beans provide fiber and minimal carbohydrates. This meal has negligible impact on blood sugar and provides excellent satiety.

Best Training-Day Pairing: Ideal for rest days or light activity days due to low carbohydrate content. For moderate to high training days, add roasted potatoes, quinoa, or a side of rice to increase carbohydrates. The lean protein makes this excellent post-workout when paired with a carbohydrate source. Simple, clean, and effective for muscle recovery.

Substitutions:

- Replace chicken breast with chicken thighs, pork tenderloin, or white fish.

- Use asparagus, broccoli, or Brussels sprouts instead of green beans.

- Add cherry tomatoes or bell peppers for additional vegetables and color.

- Use fresh thyme or rosemary instead of oregano.

- Add Parmesan cheese for additional flavor and fat.

Storage & Meal Prep Tips: This meal stores well for up to 3 days in the refrigerator. Let cool completely and store in airtight containers. Reheat in a 350°F oven for 10 to 12 minutes or in the microwave. Chicken breast can dry out when reheated, so consider adding a splash of broth or water and covering during reheating. For meal prep, cook multiple chicken breasts at once and use throughout the week in different dishes. Green beans can be batch-roasted and added to various meals.

Recipe 6: Beef and Vegetable Stir-Fry

Prep Time: 15 minutes
Cook Time: 12 minutes
Servings: 2

Ingredients:

- 12 ounces flank steak or sirloin, thinly sliced against the grain

- 2 cups broccoli florets

- 1 red bell pepper, sliced

- 1 cup snap peas

- 1 cup mushrooms, sliced

- 2 garlic cloves, minced

- 1 tablespoon fresh ginger, grated

- 3 tablespoons low-sodium soy sauce or coconut aminos

- 1 tablespoon rice vinegar

- 1 teaspoon sesame oil

- 2 tablespoons avocado oil, divided

- 1 teaspoon arrowroot powder or cornstarch

- 2 green onions, sliced

- 1 tablespoon sesame seeds

- Optional: 1 cup cooked brown rice or cauliflower rice per serving

Instructions:

1. In a small bowl, whisk together soy sauce, rice vinegar, sesame oil, and arrowroot powder. Set aside.

2. Heat 1 tablespoon of avocado oil in a large skillet or wok over high heat.

3. Add sliced beef in a single layer. Cook without stirring for 2 minutes until browned. Flip and cook for another 1 to 2 minutes. Remove beef from skillet and set aside.

4. Add remaining 1 tablespoon of avocado oil to the skillet. Add broccoli, bell pepper, snap peas, and mushrooms. Stir-fry for 4 to 5 minutes until vegetables are tender-crisp. Add a splash of water if vegetables begin to stick.

5. Add minced garlic and grated ginger. Cook for 30 seconds until fragrant.

6. Return beef to the skillet with any accumulated juices.

7. Pour sauce over beef and vegetables. Toss to coat everything evenly. Cook for 1 to 2 minutes until sauce thickens.

8. Remove from heat.

9. Divide between two bowls. If using, add cooked rice or cauliflower rice to each bowl.

10. Garnish with sliced green onions and sesame seeds.

Macronutrient Focus: High protein (approximately 38 grams), moderate fat (approximately 18 grams), low to moderate carbohydrate (approximately 16 grams without rice, 44 grams with brown rice). A protein-focused meal that scales with training needs.

Blood Sugar Impact: Low without rice, moderate with rice. The high protein and vegetables create stable blood sugar. Brown rice adds carbohydrates but remains balanced. This meal provides sustained energy without crashes.

Best Training-Day Pairing: Without rice, ideal for rest days or light activity days. With brown rice, excellent for moderate to high training days, particularly after strength training. The iron and protein from beef support muscle recovery and hormone health. The colorful vegetables provide antioxidants that reduce inflammation.

Substitutions:

- Replace beef with chicken, shrimp, tofu, or tempeh.

- Use any combination of vegetables: bok choy, carrots, zucchini, or cabbage.

- Replace brown rice with quinoa, noodles, or sweet potato.

- Use tamari for gluten-free version.

- Add cashews or peanuts for additional healthy fats and crunch.

- Replace sesame oil with chili oil for heat.

Storage & Meal Prep Tips: Stir-fry is best fresh but can be stored for up to 3 days in the refrigerator. Let cool completely and store in airtight containers. Store rice separately to prevent it from absorbing too much sauce and becoming mushy. Reheat in a skillet over medium heat or in the microwave. Add a splash of water or broth to prevent drying. For meal prep, prep all ingredients in advance and stir-fry fresh each night (takes only 10 to 12 minutes with prepped ingredients).

Recipe 7: Mediterranean Baked Cod with Tomatoes and Olives

Prep Time: 10 minutes
Cook Time: 20 minutes
Servings: 2

Ingredients:

- 2 cod fillets (6 ounces each)

- 2 cups cherry tomatoes, halved

- ½ cup Kalamata olives, pitted and halved

- ¼ cup red onion, thinly sliced

- 3 garlic cloves, minced

- 3 tablespoons olive oil

- 1 teaspoon dried oregano

- ½ teaspoon red pepper flakes (optional)

- Salt and black pepper to taste

- ¼ cup fresh basil, chopped

- 1 lemon, cut into wedges

- Optional: crumbled feta cheese

Instructions:

1. Preheat oven to 400°F (200°C).

2. In a medium bowl, combine cherry tomatoes, olives, red onion, minced garlic, 2 tablespoons of olive oil, oregano, red pepper flakes if using, salt, and pepper. Toss to combine.

3. Spread the tomato mixture in a baking dish large enough to hold both cod fillets.

4. Pat cod fillets dry with paper towels. Rub with remaining 1 tablespoon of olive oil and season with salt and pepper.

5. Place cod fillets on top of the tomato mixture.

6. Bake for 15 to 20 minutes until cod flakes easily with a fork and tomatoes are bursting and caramelized.

7. Remove from oven and let rest for 2 minutes.

8. Sprinkle with fresh basil and optional crumbled feta.

9. Serve with lemon wedges for squeezing over the fish.

Macronutrient Focus: High protein (approximately 34 grams), moderate fat (approximately 18 grams), low carbohydrate (approximately 12 grams). This is a lean, Mediterranean-inspired meal with healthy fats from olive oil and olives.

Blood Sugar Impact: Minimal. Cod provides lean protein with no carbohydrates. Tomatoes and olives provide minimal carbohydrates with fiber. This meal has negligible blood sugar impact and provides excellent satiety.

Best Training-Day Pairing: Ideal for rest days or light activity days. For moderate to high training days, serve with quinoa, couscous, or crusty whole grain bread to increase carbohydrates. The Mediterranean fats and antioxidants from tomatoes and olives reduce inflammation and support recovery. Excellent after any training session.

Substitutions:

- Replace cod with halibut, sea bass, chicken breast, or shrimp.

- Use sun-dried tomatoes instead of fresh for more concentrated flavor.

- Add artichoke hearts, capers, or roasted red peppers.

- Use fresh thyme or parsley instead of basil.

- Add spinach or kale during the last 5 minutes of baking.

Storage & Meal Prep Tips: This meal is best fresh, but leftovers can be stored in the refrigerator for up to 2 days. Reheat gently in a 350°F oven or serve cold. Cod is delicate and can dry out when reheated, so be careful not to overcook initially. The tomato and olive mixture can be made ahead and stored for up to 3 days, then reheated with fresh fish placed on top. For meal prep, make extra tomato mixture to use with different proteins throughout the week.

Recipe 8: Slow Cooker Beef and Vegetable Stew

Prep Time: 20 minutes
Cook Time: 6-8 hours (slow cooker) or 2 hours (stovetop)
Servings: 6

Ingredients:

- 2 pounds beef chuck roast, cut into 1-inch cubes

- 4 carrots, peeled and cut into chunks

- 3 celery stalks, cut into chunks

- 2 parsnips, peeled and cut into chunks

- 1 large onion, diced

- 3 garlic cloves, minced

- 2 cups mushrooms, quartered

- 1 can (14.5 ounces) diced tomatoes

- 3 cups low-sodium beef broth

- 2 tablespoons tomato paste

- 2 bay leaves

- 1 teaspoon dried thyme

- 1 teaspoon dried rosemary

- 2 tablespoons olive oil

- 2 tablespoons arrowroot powder or cornstarch (optional, for thickening)

- Salt and black pepper to taste

- Fresh parsley for garnish

Instructions:

For Slow Cooker:

1. Heat olive oil in a large skillet over high heat. Season beef cubes with salt and pepper.

2. Sear beef in batches, browning on all sides, about 2 to 3 minutes per batch. Transfer browned beef to slow cooker.

3. Add carrots, celery, parsnips, onion, garlic, and mushrooms to the slow cooker.

4. Add diced tomatoes, beef broth, tomato paste, bay leaves, thyme, and rosemary. Stir to combine.

5. Cover and cook on low for 6 to 8 hours or on high for 4 to 5 hours until beef is tender and vegetables are cooked through.

6. If you want a thicker stew, mix arrowroot powder with 2 tablespoons of cold water. Stir into stew during the last 30 minutes of cooking.

7. Remove bay leaves. Taste and adjust seasoning.

8. Serve hot, garnished with fresh parsley.

For Stovetop:

1. Follow steps 1-4 above, but use a large Dutch oven or heavy pot.

2. Bring to a boil, then reduce heat to low. Cover and simmer for 1.5 to 2 hours until beef is tender.

3. Add arrowroot slurry if desired for thickening, and cook for an additional 10 minutes.

Macronutrient Focus: High protein (approximately 32 grams per serving), moderate fat (approximately 14 grams), moderate carbohydrate (approximately 18 grams). This is a hearty, balanced meal with protein from beef and nutrients from vegetables.

Blood Sugar Impact: Low to moderate. Root vegetables provide some carbohydrates, but fiber slows absorption. The high protein and fat from beef create excellent satiety and stable blood sugar. This stew provides sustained warmth and energy for 5 to 6 hours.

Best Training-Day Pairing: Suitable for moderate training days or as a recovery meal after strength training. The carbohydrates from vegetables support glycogen replenishment. The protein and collagen from beef support muscle and connective tissue recovery. Also excellent for rest days. This is comfort food that supports longevity goals.

Substitutions:

- Replace beef chuck with lamb, venison, or boneless chicken thighs.

- Add potatoes or sweet potatoes for additional carbohydrates on heavy training days.

- Use turnips, rutabaga, or butternut squash instead of parsnips.

- Add green beans or peas during the last 30 minutes of cooking.

- Make it in an Instant Pot: pressure cook on high for 35 minutes, then natural release.

Storage & Meal Prep Tips: This stew is ideal for meal prep and tastes even better the next day. Let cool completely and store in airtight containers in the refrigerator for up to 5 days or freeze for up to 4 months. The stew will thicken as it sits; add water or broth when reheating. Reheat on the stovetop or in the microwave. Freeze in individual portions for easy grab-and-go meals. This is the ultimate make-ahead dinner that provides multiple meals throughout the week.

Recipe 9: Sheet Pan Sausage and Vegetables

Prep Time: 10 minutes
Cook Time: 30 minutes
Servings: 2

Ingredients:

- 4 chicken or turkey sausages (look for versions with minimal additives)

- 2 cups Brussels sprouts, halved

- 1 red bell pepper, cut into chunks

- 1 yellow bell pepper, cut into chunks

- 1 red onion, cut into wedges

- 1 cup cherry tomatoes

- 3 tablespoons olive oil

- 2 teaspoons Italian seasoning

- 1 teaspoon smoked paprika

- Salt and black pepper to taste

- Optional: whole grain mustard for serving

Instructions:

1. Preheat oven to 425°F (220°C). Line a large baking sheet with parchment paper.

2. Place Brussels sprouts, bell peppers, red onion, and cherry tomatoes on the baking sheet. Drizzle with olive oil, sprinkle with Italian seasoning, smoked paprika, salt, and pepper. Toss to coat evenly.

3. Arrange vegetables in a single layer, leaving space for sausages.

4. Place sausages on the baking sheet among the vegetables.

5. Roast for 25 to 30 minutes until sausages are browned and cooked through (internal temperature of 165°F) and vegetables are tender and caramelized. Flip sausages halfway through cooking.

6. Remove from oven and let rest for 5 minutes.

7. Divide sausages and vegetables between two plates.

8. Serve with optional whole grain mustard.

Macronutrient Focus: High protein (approximately 26 grams), moderate fat (approximately 22 grams), moderate carbohydrate (approximately 22 grams). The macronutrient profile depends on sausage type; choose lean chicken or turkey sausages for lower fat.

Blood Sugar Impact: Low to moderate. Vegetables provide fiber and minimal carbohydrates. The protein and fat from sausages create stable blood sugar. This meal provides sustained energy and satiety.

Best Training-Day Pairing: Suitable for moderate training days or rest days depending on sausage choice and portion size. For heavy training days, add roasted potatoes or serve with brown rice. The convenience and flavor make this an excellent weeknight option when time is limited.

Substitutions:

- Replace chicken sausage with pork sausage, beef sausage, or plant-based sausage.

- Use any combination of vegetables: zucchini, broccoli, cauliflower, or sweet potatoes.

- Add fennel, eggplant, or mushrooms for variety.

- Season with different spice blends: Cajun, Greek, or curry powder.

- Add chickpeas or white beans for additional protein and fiber.

Storage & Meal Prep Tips: This sheet pan meal stores well for up to 4 days in the refrigerator. Let cool completely and store in airtight containers. Reheat in a 350°F oven for 10 to 12 minutes or in the microwave. For meal prep, this is one of the simplest approaches: everything cooks on one pan, cleanup is minimal, and the meal provides balanced nutrition. Prep vegetables in advance and store in containers, then simply arrange on the sheet pan when ready to cook.

Recipe 10: Thai-Inspired Chicken Curry

Prep Time: 15 minutes
Cook Time: 25 minutes
Servings: 4

Ingredients:

- 1.5 pounds boneless, skinless chicken thighs, cut into bite-sized pieces

- 1 can (13.5 ounces) full-fat coconut milk

- 2 tablespoons red curry paste (adjust to taste)

- 1 red bell pepper, sliced

- 1 cup green beans, trimmed and halved

- 1 cup broccoli florets

- 1 small onion, sliced

- 3 garlic cloves, minced

- 1 tablespoon fresh ginger, grated

- 1 tablespoon fish sauce (or soy sauce)

- 1 tablespoon lime juice

- 1 tablespoon coconut oil

- Fresh basil and cilantro for garnish

- Optional: 2 cups cooked jasmine rice or cauliflower rice

Instructions:

1. Heat coconut oil in a large skillet or Dutch oven over medium-high heat.

2. Add chicken pieces and cook for 5 to 6 minutes until browned on all sides. Remove chicken and set aside.

3. In the same skillet, add sliced onion. Sauté for 3 minutes until softened.

4. Add minced garlic, grated ginger, and red curry paste. Cook for 1 minute, stirring constantly, until fragrant.

5. Pour in coconut milk and stir to combine with the curry paste.

6. Add fish sauce and bring to a simmer.

7. Return chicken to the skillet. Add bell pepper, green beans, and broccoli.

8. Reduce heat to medium-low and simmer for 12 to 15 minutes until chicken is cooked through and vegetables are tender.

9. Stir in lime juice.

10. Taste and adjust seasoning. Add more curry paste for heat or fish sauce for saltiness.

11. Serve over optional rice or cauliflower rice.

12. Garnish with fresh basil and cilantro.

Macronutrient Focus: High protein (approximately 34 grams per serving), moderate to high fat (approximately 24 grams from coconut milk), moderate carbohydrate (approximately 16 grams without rice, 50 grams with jasmine rice). The coconut milk provides healthy saturated fats.

Blood Sugar Impact: Low without rice, moderate with rice. The protein and fat from chicken and coconut milk create stable blood sugar. The vegetables add fiber. Jasmine rice adds carbohydrates but remains balanced in the context of this meal.

Best Training-Day Pairing: Without rice, suitable for rest days or light activity days. With jasmine rice, excellent for moderate to high training days, particularly after strength training or cardio. The curry flavors and coconut milk make this a satisfying, warming meal that supports recovery.

Substitutions:

- Replace chicken with shrimp, tofu, or white fish (reduce cooking time accordingly).

- Use any vegetables: snap peas, carrots, zucchini, mushrooms, or spinach.

- Replace red curry paste with green or yellow curry paste for different flavor profiles.

- Use light coconut milk to reduce fat and calories.

- Add bamboo shoots or water chestnuts for texture.

- Replace fish sauce with soy sauce or coconut aminos.

Storage & Meal Prep Tips: This curry stores exceptionally well and tastes even better the next day as flavors meld. Let cool completely and store in airtight containers in the refrigerator for up to 4 days or freeze for up to 3 months. Store rice separately to prevent it from becoming mushy. Reheat on the stovetop or in the microwave, adding a splash of coconut milk or water if needed. This is an excellent meal prep option that provides multiple servings with minimal effort.

Recipe 11: Pork Tenderloin with Roasted Brussels Sprouts and Apple

Prep Time: 15 minutes
Cook Time: 30 minutes
Servings: 4

Ingredients:

- 1.5 pounds pork tenderloin

- 1 pound Brussels sprouts, halved

- 2 medium apples, cored and cut into wedges

- 1 red onion, cut into wedges

- 4 tablespoons olive oil, divided

- 2 tablespoons balsamic vinegar

- 2 tablespoons Dijon mustard

- 2 garlic cloves, minced

- 1 teaspoon dried thyme

- 1 teaspoon dried rosemary

- Salt and black pepper to taste

Instructions:

1. Preheat oven to 425°F (220°C). Line a large baking sheet with parchment paper.

2. Pat pork tenderloin dry with paper towels. Season all sides with thyme, rosemary, salt, and pepper.

3. In a small bowl, mix together 2 tablespoons of olive oil, balsamic vinegar, Dijon mustard, and minced garlic to create a glaze.

4. Place Brussels sprouts, apple wedges, and red onion on the baking sheet. Drizzle with remaining 2 tablespoons of olive oil and season with salt and pepper. Toss to coat and spread in a single layer.

5. Push vegetables to the sides of the baking sheet and place pork tenderloin in the center.

6. Brush half of the balsamic glaze over the pork.

7. Roast for 20 minutes.

8. Remove from oven and brush pork with remaining glaze. Stir vegetables.

9. Return to oven and roast for another 8 to 10 minutes until pork reaches an internal temperature of 145°F and vegetables are caramelized.

10. Remove from oven and let pork rest for 5 to 10 minutes before slicing.

11. Slice pork into medallions and serve with roasted vegetables and apples.

Macronutrient Focus: High protein (approximately 38 grams), moderate fat (approximately 14 grams), moderate carbohydrate (approximately 24 grams). Pork tenderloin is one of the leanest cuts of meat available, comparable to chicken breast.

Blood Sugar Impact: Low to moderate. Apples add natural sweetness and carbohydrates, but their fiber content and the high protein from pork create a balanced blood sugar response. Brussels sprouts add additional fiber. This meal provides sustained energy without spikes.

Best Training-Day Pairing: Suitable for moderate training days or as a recovery meal after strength training or Zone 2 cardio. The carbohydrates from apples provide some fuel without being excessive. Also excellent for rest days. The combination of savory and sweet makes this a satisfying, complete meal.

Substitutions:

- Replace pork with chicken breast or salmon.

- Use pears instead of apples for a different fruit profile.

- Replace Brussels sprouts with broccoli, cauliflower, or butternut squash.

- Add sweet potatoes for additional carbohydrates on heavy training days.

- Use honey instead of balsamic vinegar for a sweeter glaze.

- Add pecans or walnuts during the last 5 minutes of roasting for healthy fats and crunch.

Storage & Meal Prep Tips: This meal stores well for up to 4 days in the refrigerator. Let cool completely and store in airtight containers. Pork tenderloin can dry out when reheated, so add a splash of broth or water and cover during reheating. Reheat in a 350°F oven for 10 to 12 minutes or in the microwave. Slice leftover pork and use in salads, wraps, or grain bowls throughout the week. The roasted vegetables reheat well and maintain good texture.

Recipe 12: Shrimp Scampi with Zucchini Noodles

Prep Time: 10 minutes
Cook Time: 10 minutes
Servings: 2

Ingredients:

- 1 pound large shrimp, peeled and deveined

- 3 medium zucchini, spiralized into noodles

- 4 garlic cloves, minced

- ¼ cup dry white wine (or chicken broth)

- 2 tablespoons lemon juice

- 3 tablespoons olive oil, divided

- 2 tablespoons butter (or ghee)

- ¼ teaspoon red pepper flakes

- Salt and black pepper to taste

- ¼ cup fresh parsley, chopped

- Lemon wedges for serving

- Optional: grated Parmesan cheese

Instructions:

1. Pat shrimp dry with paper towels and season with salt and pepper.

2. Heat 2 tablespoons of olive oil in a large skillet over medium-high heat.

3. Add shrimp in a single layer and cook for 2 minutes per side until pink and opaque. Remove shrimp from skillet and set aside.

4. In the same skillet, reduce heat to medium and add butter. Once melted, add minced garlic and red pepper flakes. Cook for 30 seconds until fragrant (don't let garlic burn).

5. Add white wine (or broth) and lemon juice. Bring to a simmer and cook for 2 minutes to reduce slightly.

6. Add zucchini noodles to the skillet. Toss with tongs for 2 to 3 minutes until just tender (don't overcook or they'll become watery).

7. Return shrimp to the skillet with any accumulated juices. Toss everything together for 1 minute to heat through.

8. Remove from heat and stir in remaining 1 tablespoon of olive oil and chopped parsley.

114

9. Divide between two bowls or plates.

10. Serve with lemon wedges and optional Parmesan cheese.

Macronutrient Focus: High protein (approximately 42 grams), moderate fat (approximately 20 grams), low carbohydrate (approximately 10 grams). This is a lean, low-carb meal that's quick to prepare.

Blood Sugar Impact: Minimal. Shrimp provides lean protein with virtually no carbohydrates. Zucchini noodles are very low in carbohydrates compared to pasta. This meal has negligible blood sugar impact and provides excellent satiety.

Best Training-Day Pairing: Ideal for rest days or light activity days due to low carbohydrate content. For moderate to high training days, serve with whole grain pasta alongside or instead of zucchini noodles, or add a side of roasted potatoes. The lean protein from shrimp supports muscle recovery without excess calories. This is also excellent for post-workout when paired with a carbohydrate source.

Substitutions:

- Replace shrimp with scallops, chicken breast, or white fish.

- Use regular spaghetti, linguine, or angel hair pasta instead of zucchini noodles for higher carbohydrates.

- Use spaghetti squash as another low-carb alternative to pasta.

- Replace white wine with additional broth plus a splash of vinegar.

- Add cherry tomatoes or spinach for additional vegetables.

- Make it dairy-free by using only olive oil (omit butter and Parmesan).

Storage & Meal Prep Tips: This dish is best fresh, as shrimp and zucchini noodles both lose texture when stored and reheated. If you must make ahead, cook the shrimp and store separately. Spiralize zucchini and store raw in a container lined with paper towels for up to 2 days. Sauté the zucchini noodles and reheat the shrimp together just before serving. This meal comes together so quickly (10 minutes) that it's best to make fresh rather than meal prep.

Recipe 13: Chicken Fajita Bowl

Prep Time: 15 minutes
Cook Time: 20 minutes
Servings: 2

Ingredients:

For Chicken:

- 12 ounces boneless, skinless chicken breast, sliced into strips

- 1 tablespoon olive oil

- 1 teaspoon chili powder

- 1 teaspoon cumin

- 1 teaspoon paprika

- ½ teaspoon garlic powder

- Salt and black pepper to taste

For Vegetables:

- 1 red bell pepper, sliced

- 1 yellow bell pepper, sliced

- 1 green bell pepper, sliced

- 1 large onion, sliced

- 1 tablespoon olive oil

For Bowl:

- 2 cups cooked brown rice, cilantro-lime rice, or cauliflower rice

- 1 avocado, sliced

- ½ cup black beans, drained and rinsed

- ¼ cup salsa

- ¼ cup Greek yogurt or sour cream

- ¼ cup shredded cheese (cheddar or Mexican blend)

- 2 tablespoons fresh cilantro, chopped

- 1 lime, cut into wedges

Instructions:

1. In a medium bowl, toss chicken strips with chili powder, cumin, paprika, garlic powder, salt, and pepper.

2. Heat 1 tablespoon of olive oil in a large skillet over medium-high heat.

3. Add seasoned chicken and cook for 6 to 8 minutes, stirring occasionally, until cooked through and lightly charred. Remove chicken from skillet and set aside.

4. In the same skillet, add 1 tablespoon of olive oil. Add sliced bell peppers and onion. Cook for 6 to 8 minutes, stirring occasionally, until vegetables are tender and slightly caramelized. Season with salt and pepper.

5. Divide rice or cauliflower rice between two bowls.

6. Top each bowl with cooked chicken, sautéed peppers and onions, black beans, avocado slices, salsa, Greek yogurt, and shredded cheese.

7. Garnish with fresh cilantro and serve with lime wedges.

Macronutrient Focus: High protein (approximately 44 grams with brown rice, 48 grams with cauliflower rice), moderate fat (approximately 22 grams), moderate carbohydrate (approximately 52 grams with brown rice, 28 grams with cauliflower rice). This is a customizable, balanced meal.

Blood Sugar Impact: Moderate with brown rice, low with cauliflower rice. The high protein from chicken and beans, combined with fiber from vegetables and beans, creates stable blood sugar. Brown rice adds carbohydrates but remains balanced. Cauliflower rice version has minimal blood sugar impact.

Best Training-Day Pairing: With brown rice, excellent for moderate to high training days, particularly after strength training or intense cardio. The carbohydrates support glycogen replenishment and the protein supports muscle recovery. With cauliflower rice, ideal for rest days or light activity days. This bowl is versatile and satisfying regardless of training schedule.

Substitutions:

- Replace chicken with steak, shrimp, or grilled tofu.
- Use quinoa, wild rice, or sweet potato instead of brown rice.
- Replace black beans with pinto beans or refried beans.
- Add corn for additional carbohydrates and sweetness.
- Use full sour cream instead of Greek yogurt if preferred.
- Make it dairy-free by omitting cheese and using coconut yogurt.
- Add jalapeños or hot sauce for additional heat.

Storage & Meal Prep Tips: This bowl is excellent for meal prep. Cook chicken, peppers and onions, rice, and beans separately. Store in individual containers in the refrigerator for up to 4 days. Assemble bowls fresh each day with toppings like avocado, salsa, and Greek yogurt. This prevents ingredients from becoming soggy and allows you to customize each bowl. Reheat the cooked components separately or together in the microwave or on the stovetop. Add fresh toppings just before eating.

Recipe 14: Baked Eggplant Parmesan (Lighter Version)

Prep Time: 20 minutes
Cook Time: 35 minutes
Servings: 4

Ingredients:

- 2 large eggplants, sliced into ½-inch rounds

- 2 cups marinara sauce (look for low-sugar versions)

- 1½ cups shredded mozzarella cheese

- ½ cup grated Parmesan cheese

- 1 cup almond flour or whole wheat breadcrumbs

- 2 eggs, beaten

- 2 tablespoons olive oil

- 2 teaspoons Italian seasoning

- 1 teaspoon garlic powder

- Salt and black pepper to taste

- Fresh basil for garnish

- Optional: side salad or whole grain pasta

Instructions:

1. Preheat oven to 400°F (200°C). Line two baking sheets with parchment paper and brush lightly with olive oil.

2. Arrange eggplant slices on paper towels and sprinkle both sides with salt. Let sit for 10 minutes to draw out moisture. Pat dry with paper towels.

3. In a shallow bowl, beat eggs with 1 tablespoon of water.

4. In another shallow bowl, combine almond flour (or breadcrumbs), Italian seasoning, garlic powder, salt, and pepper.

5. Dip each eggplant slice in beaten egg, then coat in the almond flour mixture, pressing to adhere. Place on prepared baking sheets.

6. Bake for 20 minutes, flipping halfway through, until golden and tender.

7. Reduce oven temperature to 375°F (190°C).

8. Spread ½ cup of marinara sauce in the bottom of a 9x13-inch baking dish.

9. Layer half of the baked eggplant slices over the sauce. Top with half of the remaining marinara, half of the mozzarella, and half of the Parmesan.

10. Repeat layers with remaining eggplant, marinara, and cheeses.

11. Bake for 15 to 20 minutes until cheese is melted and bubbly.

12. Let rest for 5 minutes before serving.

13. Garnish with fresh basil.

Macronutrient Focus: High protein (approximately 22 grams per serving), moderate fat (approximately 18 grams), moderate carbohydrate (approximately 28 grams). This lighter version is baked rather than fried, significantly reducing fat and calories while maintaining flavor.

Blood Sugar Impact: Low to moderate. Eggplant is very low in carbohydrates and high in fiber. The marinara sauce contains some carbohydrates from tomatoes, but the protein and fat from cheese create a balanced response. This meal provides sustained energy without spikes.

Best Training-Day Pairing: Suitable for moderate training days or rest days. For heavy training days, serve with whole grain pasta or crusty bread to increase carbohydrates. The protein from cheese supports muscle maintenance. This is a comfort food that fits longevity goals.

Substitutions:

- Replace almond flour with regular breadcrumbs, panko, or crushed pork rinds for different textures and macros.

- Use zucchini slices instead of eggplant for variety.

- Add a layer of sautéed spinach or mushrooms between eggplant layers.

- Use dairy-free mozzarella and nutritional yeast instead of Parmesan for a vegan version.

- Add ground turkey or Italian sausage between layers for additional protein.

Storage & Meal Prep Tips: Eggplant Parmesan stores exceptionally well and actually tastes better the next day as flavors meld. Let cool completely and store in airtight containers in the refrigerator for up to 4 days or freeze for up to 3 months. Reheat in a 350°F oven for 15 to 20 minutes or in the microwave. This is an excellent make-ahead dinner that provides multiple servings. You can also assemble the dish completely, cover tightly, and refrigerate for up to 24 hours before baking.

Recipe 15: Lemon Herb Grilled Chicken Thighs with Roasted Cauliflower

Prep Time: 10 minutes (plus 30 minutes marinating)
Cook Time: 25 minutes
Servings: 2

Ingredients:

For Chicken:

- 4 boneless, skinless chicken thighs

- 3 tablespoons olive oil

- 3 tablespoons lemon juice

- 2 garlic cloves, minced

- 1 tablespoon fresh rosemary, chopped (or 1 teaspoon dried)

119

- 1 tablespoon fresh thyme, chopped (or 1 teaspoon dried)

- 1 teaspoon lemon zest

- Salt and black pepper to taste

For Cauliflower:

- 1 large head cauliflower, cut into florets

- 2 tablespoons olive oil

- 2 garlic cloves, minced

- 1 teaspoon smoked paprika

- ½ teaspoon cumin

- Salt and black pepper to taste

- 2 tablespoons fresh parsley, chopped

- Optional: grated Parmesan cheese

Instructions:

1. In a medium bowl, whisk together olive oil, lemon juice, minced garlic, rosemary, thyme, lemon zest, salt, and pepper to create marinade.

2. Add chicken thighs and toss to coat. Cover and refrigerate for at least 30 minutes (up to 4 hours for more flavor).

3. Preheat oven to 425°F (220°C). Line a baking sheet with parchment paper.

4. Toss cauliflower florets with olive oil, minced garlic, smoked paprika, cumin, salt, and pepper. Spread in a single layer on the baking sheet.

5. Roast cauliflower for 25 to 30 minutes, stirring halfway through, until tender and golden brown with crispy edges.

6. While cauliflower roasts, heat a grill or grill pan over medium-high heat. If using a skillet, heat over medium-high heat.

7. Remove chicken from marinade (discard excess marinade). Grill or cook chicken for 5 to 6 minutes per side until cooked through (internal temperature of 165°F) and nicely charred.

8. Let chicken rest for 5 minutes.

9. Remove cauliflower from oven and toss with fresh parsley and optional Parmesan.

10. Divide chicken and cauliflower between two plates.

Macronutrient Focus: High protein (approximately 36 grams), moderate fat (approximately 24 grams), low carbohydrate (approximately 14 grams). Chicken thighs are slightly higher in fat than breasts but remain a lean protein source with excellent flavor.

Blood Sugar Impact: Minimal. Chicken provides protein and fat with no carbohydrates. Cauliflower is very low in carbohydrates and high in fiber. This meal has negligible blood sugar impact and provides excellent satiety.

Best Training-Day Pairing: Ideal for rest days or light activity days due to low carbohydrate content. For moderate to high training days, add roasted sweet potatoes, quinoa, or brown rice to increase carbohydrates. The protein from chicken supports muscle recovery. The herbs and lemon provide anti-inflammatory compounds. Simple, clean, and effective.

Substitutions:

- Replace chicken thighs with chicken breast, pork chops, or salmon.

- Use broccoli, Brussels sprouts, or a combination instead of cauliflower.

- Replace fresh herbs with Italian seasoning or herbs de Provence.

- Add cherry tomatoes to the cauliflower during the last 10 minutes of roasting.

- Make cauliflower "rice" by pulsing raw cauliflower in a food processor, then sautéing for 5 to 7 minutes.

Storage & Meal Prep Tips: Marinate chicken up to 24 hours in advance for maximum flavor. Cooked chicken thighs store well in the refrigerator for up to 4 days. Roasted cauliflower can be stored for up to 4 days but loses some crispness. Reheat chicken and cauliflower in a 350°F oven for 10 minutes or in the microwave. For meal prep, cook extra chicken to use in salads, wraps, or grain bowls throughout the week. The roasted cauliflower is excellent cold in salads or reheated as a side.

Recipe 16: Ground Turkey and Vegetable Skillet

Prep Time: 10 minutes
Cook Time: 20 minutes
Servings: 4

Ingredients:

- 1.5 pounds ground turkey (93% lean)

- 1 large zucchini, diced

- 1 red bell pepper, diced

- 1 yellow bell pepper, diced

- 1 cup cherry tomatoes, halved

- 1 cup mushrooms, sliced

- 1 small onion, diced

- 3 garlic cloves, minced

- 2 tablespoons olive oil

- 1 teaspoon Italian seasoning

- 1 teaspoon smoked paprika

- ½ teaspoon red pepper flakes (optional)

- Salt and black pepper to taste

- ¼ cup fresh basil, chopped

- Optional: grated Parmesan cheese and serve over zucchini noodles, pasta, or quinoa

Instructions:

1. Heat 1 tablespoon of olive oil in a large skillet over medium-high heat.

2. Add ground turkey, breaking it up with a spatula. Cook for 6 to 8 minutes until browned and cooked through. Season with salt and pepper. Remove turkey from skillet and set aside.

3. In the same skillet, add remaining 1 tablespoon of olive oil. Add diced onion and cook for 2 to 3 minutes until softened.

4. Add minced garlic, Italian seasoning, smoked paprika, and red pepper flakes if using. Cook for 30 seconds until fragrant.

5. Add diced zucchini, bell peppers, and mushrooms. Cook for 6 to 8 minutes, stirring occasionally, until vegetables are tender.

6. Add cherry tomatoes and cook for 2 to 3 minutes until they begin to soften and release juices.

7. Return cooked turkey to the skillet with any accumulated juices. Stir to combine and heat through.

8. Taste and adjust seasoning.

9. Remove from heat and stir in fresh basil.

10. Serve as is, or over optional zucchini noodles, pasta, or quinoa.

11. Top with optional Parmesan cheese.

Macronutrient Focus: High protein (approximately 32 grams per serving), low fat (approximately 10 grams), low carbohydrate (approximately 10 grams as written). Adding pasta or quinoa increases carbohydrates significantly.

Blood Sugar Impact: Minimal as written. Ground turkey provides lean protein with no carbohydrates. Vegetables provide fiber and minimal carbohydrates. This meal has very low blood sugar impact and provides excellent satiety. Adding pasta or quinoa increases blood sugar response but remains balanced due to high protein content.

Best Training-Day Pairing: As written, ideal for rest days or light activity days. For moderate to high training days, serve over pasta, quinoa, or brown rice to increase carbohydrates. The lean protein from turkey makes this excellent post-workout when paired with a carbohydrate source. This is a simple, versatile meal that can be adjusted to any training schedule.

Substitutions:

- Replace ground turkey with ground chicken, beef, or plant-based meat alternative.

- Use any combination of vegetables: eggplant, spinach, kale, or green beans.

- Replace Italian seasoning with taco seasoning for a Mexican-inspired version.

- Add white beans or chickpeas for additional fiber and carbohydrates.

- Use marinara sauce instead of cherry tomatoes for a richer, saucier dish.

Storage & Meal Prep Tips: This skillet meal is ideal for meal prep. Let cool completely and store in airtight containers in the refrigerator for up to 4 days or freeze for up to 3 months. Reheat in a skillet over medium heat or in the microwave, adding a splash of water or broth to prevent drying. The vegetables release moisture as they sit, creating a light sauce. If meal prepping with pasta or quinoa, store the turkey-vegetable mixture and grain separately to prevent the grain from absorbing too much liquid and becoming mushy.

Recipe 17: Balsamic Glazed Salmon with Roasted Vegetables

Prep Time: 10 minutes
Cook Time: 20 minutes
Servings: 2

Ingredients:

For Salmon:

- 2 salmon fillets (6 ounces each)

- 2 tablespoons balsamic vinegar

- 1 tablespoon honey

- 1 tablespoon Dijon mustard

- 2 garlic cloves, minced

- 1 tablespoon olive oil

- Salt and black pepper to taste

For Vegetables:

- 2 cups broccoli florets

- 1 red bell pepper, cut into chunks

- 1 cup cherry tomatoes

- 1 small red onion, cut into wedges

- 2 tablespoons olive oil

- 1 teaspoon dried thyme

- Salt and black pepper to taste

Instructions:

1. Preheat oven to 400°F (200°C). Line a large baking sheet with parchment paper.

2. In a small bowl, whisk together balsamic vinegar, honey, Dijon mustard, and minced garlic to create the glaze.

3. Place broccoli, bell pepper, cherry tomatoes, and red onion on one side of the baking sheet. Drizzle with olive oil, sprinkle with thyme, salt, and pepper. Toss to coat.

4. Pat salmon fillets dry with paper towels. Rub with olive oil and season with salt and pepper. Place salmon on the other side of the baking sheet.

5. Brush salmon generously with half of the balsamic glaze.

6. Roast for 12 minutes.

7. Remove from oven and brush salmon with remaining glaze.

8. Return to oven and roast for another 5 to 8 minutes until salmon flakes easily with a fork and vegetables are tender and caramelized.

9. Divide salmon and vegetables between two plates.

Macronutrient Focus: High protein (approximately 38 grams), moderate fat (approximately 22 grams, mostly omega-3s), moderate carbohydrate (approximately 18 grams). The honey adds minimal carbohydrates but creates a delicious glaze.

Blood Sugar Impact: Low to moderate. Salmon provides protein and omega-3 fatty acids with no carbohydrates. Vegetables provide fiber and minimal carbohydrates. The small amount of honey in the glaze has minimal blood sugar impact in the context of this high-protein meal.

Best Training-Day Pairing: Suitable for rest days or light to moderate activity days. For heavy training days, add quinoa, sweet potato, or brown rice to increase carbohydrates. The omega-3s from salmon reduce inflammation and support recovery, making this excellent after any training session. The balsamic glaze adds flavor without significantly impacting nutrition.

Substitutions:

- Replace salmon with chicken breast, pork tenderloin, or tofu.

- Use any vegetables: zucchini, asparagus, cauliflower, or Brussels sprouts.

- Replace honey with maple syrup or omit for lower carbohydrates.

- Add green beans or snap peas for additional vegetables.

- Use fresh rosemary instead of thyme for different flavor.

Storage & Meal Prep Tips: This meal is best fresh, but leftovers can be stored in the refrigerator for up to 2 days. Salmon is delicate and can dry out when reheated, so be gentle. Reheat in a 350°F oven for 8 to 10 minutes or serve cold on salads. The roasted vegetables reheat well and maintain good texture. For meal prep, make extra glaze to use on different proteins throughout the week. Cook extra vegetables to use as sides with various meals.

Recipe 18: Moroccan-Spiced Chicken with Roasted Carrots and Chickpeas

Prep Time: 15 minutes
Cook Time: 35 minutes
Servings: 4

Ingredients:

For Chicken:

- 1.5 pounds boneless, skinless chicken thighs

- 2 tablespoons olive oil

- 2 teaspoons cumin

- 2 teaspoons coriander

- 1 teaspoon cinnamon

- 1 teaspoon smoked paprika

- ½ teaspoon turmeric

- ½ teaspoon cayenne pepper (optional)

- Salt and black pepper to taste

For Vegetables and Chickpeas:

- 1 can (15 ounces) chickpeas, drained and rinsed

- 1 pound carrots, peeled and cut into chunks

- 1 red onion, cut into wedges

- 2 tablespoons olive oil

- 1 teaspoon cumin

- Salt and black pepper to taste

For Serving:

- ¼ cup fresh cilantro, chopped

- ¼ cup fresh mint, chopped

- ¼ cup Greek yogurt or tahini sauce

- Lemon wedges

- Optional: couscous or cauliflower rice

Instructions:

1. Preheat oven to 425°F (220°C). Line a large baking sheet with parchment paper.

2. In a small bowl, combine cumin, coriander, cinnamon, smoked paprika, turmeric, cayenne if using, salt, and pepper to create spice mix.

3. Pat chicken thighs dry with paper towels. Rub with 1 tablespoon of olive oil, then coat generously with the spice mix on both sides.

4. In a large bowl, toss chickpeas, carrots, and red onion with 2 tablespoons of olive oil, 1 teaspoon cumin, salt, and pepper.

5. Spread vegetables and chickpeas on the baking sheet. Place seasoned chicken thighs on top.

6. Drizzle chicken with remaining 1 tablespoon of olive oil.

7. Roast for 30 to 35 minutes until chicken is cooked through (internal temperature of 165°F) and vegetables are tender and caramelized.

8. Remove from oven and let rest for 5 minutes.

9. Transfer chicken, vegetables, and chickpeas to a serving platter.

10. Top with chopped cilantro and mint.

11. Serve with Greek yogurt or tahini sauce and lemon wedges.

12. Add optional couscous or cauliflower rice as a base.

Macronutrient Focus: High protein (approximately 38 grams per serving), moderate fat (approximately 18 grams), moderate carbohydrate (approximately 28 grams). Chickpeas provide both protein and carbohydrates along with significant fiber.

Blood Sugar Impact: Low to moderate. Chickpeas are high in fiber and protein, which significantly slow glucose absorption. The carrots add natural sweetness and carbohydrates, but fiber slows absorption. Combined with the high protein from chicken, this meal produces stable blood sugar and sustained energy.

Best Training-Day Pairing: Excellent for moderate to high training days, particularly after strength training or cardio. The carbohydrates from chickpeas and carrots support glycogen replenishment. The protein supports muscle recovery. Also suitable for rest days due to the balanced macronutrient profile. The warming spices have anti-inflammatory properties.

Substitutions:

- Replace chicken thighs with chicken breast, lamb, or tofu.

- Use sweet potatoes instead of carrots for different nutrients and sweetness.

- Add cauliflower florets for additional vegetables.

- Replace chickpeas with white beans or lentils.

- Use parsley instead of cilantro if you prefer.

- Make a yogurt-tahini sauce by mixing equal parts Greek yogurt and tahini with lemon juice and garlic.

Storage & Meal Prep Tips: This Moroccan-inspired dish is excellent for meal prep and tastes even better the next day as flavors meld. Let cool completely and store in airtight containers in the refrigerator for up to 4 days or freeze for up to 3 months. Reheat in a 350°F oven for 15 minutes or in the microwave. Store the yogurt or tahini sauce separately and add fresh herbs just before serving. This is a flavorful, satisfying meal that provides multiple servings with minimal effort.

[CHAPTER INTEGRATION]

These eighteen dinner recipes provide substantial variety while maintaining the core nutritional principles that support longevity. Each recipe prioritizes protein for muscle maintenance and recovery, includes vegetables for fiber and micronutrients, and offers flexibility with carbohydrate content based on training demands.

The recipes span multiple cuisines and cooking methods: sheet pan meals for convenience, slow cooker options for hands-off cooking, quick skillet dinners for busy weeknights, and more involved preparations for when you have time. Several are ideal for meal prep, allowing you to cook once and enjoy multiple meals throughout the week.

Notice that each recipe can be adjusted to match your training schedule. Lower-carbohydrate versions work for rest days or light activity days. Adding grains, potatoes, or other carbohydrate sources transforms the same base recipe into a meal suitable for heavy training days. This flexibility is key to sustainable nutrition.

As with breakfast and lunch, these are templates, not rigid prescriptions. Adjust portions based on your body size, activity level, and training schedule. Swap ingredients based on preferences, dietary restrictions, or what you have available. The principles remain constant: build meals around protein, include plenty of vegetables, choose quality carbohydrates when needed, and incorporate healthy fats.

Pay attention to how these meals make you feel. Do they keep you satisfied until bedtime without late-night snacking? Do you wake up feeling recovered and ready for the next day? Are you maintaining energy throughout your training sessions? Use this feedback to adjust portions and macronutrient ratios.

Dinner is not just about eating. It is about recovery, restoration, and preparation for tomorrow. When you end the day with a protein-rich, nutrient-dense meal, you support overnight muscle repair, hormone production, and metabolic health. You set yourself up for better sleep, better recovery, and better performance the next day.

Make dinner a priority. Plan it. Prepare it. Enjoy it. Your body will thank you for decades.

CHAPTER 10: SNACKS & RECOVERY MEALS

Snacking has become one of the most misunderstood aspects of nutrition. The food industry has convinced us that we need to eat constantly, grazing throughout the day to "keep our metabolism going" or "prevent hunger." Meanwhile, most snack foods are engineered to be hyper-palatable, nutritionally empty, and impossible to eat in moderation.

The truth is more nuanced. Strategic snacking, when done correctly, can support training, prevent excessive hunger between meals, and provide convenient nutrition when needed. But mindless snacking, driven by boredom, stress, or habit rather than genuine hunger, undermines metabolic health and body composition.

This chapter focuses on snacks and recovery meals that serve a purpose. These are not convenience foods to be eaten mindlessly while watching television. They are strategic nutrition tools designed to support training, bridge gaps between meals when needed, and provide immediate post-workout recovery nutrition.

Recovery meals deserve special attention. The period immediately following training, particularly intense strength training or high-intensity cardio, is when your body is most receptive to nutrients. Consuming protein and carbohydrates within one to two hours after training supports muscle protein synthesis, glycogen replenishment, and recovery processes that determine how well you adapt to training.

This chapter provides ten snack and recovery meal options. Each recipe includes timing information, macronutrient focus, best use cases, and preparation guidance. Some are designed for post-workout recovery. Others work as pre-workout fuel or as strategic snacks between meals. All are built around whole foods and support your longevity goals.

Let's be clear about when to use these recipes: when you are genuinely hungry between meals, when you need fuel before or after training, or when your schedule requires eating at unconventional times. Not when you are bored, stressed, or eating out of habit.

Let's begin.

Recipe 1: Post-Workout Recovery Smoothie

Prep Time: 5 minutes
Cook Time: 0 minutes
Servings: 1

Ingredients:

- 1 scoop vanilla or chocolate protein powder (whey or plant-based, approximately 20-25g protein)

- 1 cup unsweetened almond milk or milk of choice

- 1 frozen banana

- ½ cup frozen berries (mixed or blueberries)

- 1 tablespoon almond butter or peanut butter

- 1 tablespoon ground flaxseed

- ½ cup ice cubes

- Optional: 1 tablespoon honey for additional carbohydrates

Instructions:

1. Add all ingredients to a high-speed blender in the order listed (liquid first helps blending).

2. Blend on high for 45 to 60 seconds until completely smooth and creamy.

3. Check consistency. If too thick, add more liquid. If too thin, add more ice or frozen fruit.

4. Pour into a glass and consume immediately.

Macronutrient Focus: High protein (approximately 32 grams), moderate fat (approximately 12 grams), moderate to high carbohydrate (approximately 45 grams, 52 grams with honey). This is a complete recovery meal in liquid form.

Blood Sugar Impact: Moderate. The protein powder and nut butter provide substantial protein and fat that slow the absorption of carbohydrates from fruit. While the banana and berries contain natural sugars, the overall blood sugar response remains moderate and appropriate for post-workout recovery.

Best Use Case: Consume within 30 to 60 minutes after strength training or high-intensity cardio when your body is primed for nutrient uptake. The combination of fast-digesting protein and carbohydrates supports muscle protein synthesis and glycogen replenishment. This is particularly useful when you cannot eat a full meal immediately after training. Also suitable as a quick breakfast when time is limited.

Substitutions:

- Replace frozen banana with ½ cup cooked oatmeal for different carbohydrates and texture.

- Use any frozen fruit: mango, pineapple, cherries, or peaches.

- Replace nut butter with ¼ avocado for healthy fats.

- Add 1 cup fresh spinach for additional micronutrients (you won't taste it).

- Use Greek yogurt instead of protein powder for a creamier texture (adjust liquid accordingly).

- Add collagen peptides for additional protein and joint support.

Storage & Meal Prep Tips: Smoothies are best consumed immediately after blending, but you can prep freezer packs for convenience. Place all ingredients except liquid and protein powder into individual freezer bags or containers. In the morning or post-workout, dump the frozen contents into the blender, add liquid and protein powder, and blend. Blended smoothies can be stored in the refrigerator for up to 24 hours in an airtight bottle or jar. Shake well before drinking as separation is normal.

Recipe 2: Hard-Boiled Eggs with Avocado and Everything Seasoning

Prep Time: 2 minutes (eggs pre-cooked)
Cook Time: 0 minutes
Servings: 1

Ingredients:

- 2-3 hard-boiled eggs, peeled

- ½ avocado, sliced

- 1 teaspoon everything bagel seasoning

- ¼ teaspoon red pepper flakes (optional)

- Salt and black pepper to taste

- Optional: cherry tomatoes or cucumber slices

Instructions:

1. Slice hard-boiled eggs in half lengthwise.

2. Arrange egg halves and avocado slices on a plate.

3. Sprinkle with everything bagel seasoning, red pepper flakes if using, salt, and pepper.

4. Add optional cherry tomatoes or cucumber slices for additional volume and nutrients.

5. Eat immediately.

Macronutrient Focus: High protein (approximately 18 grams with 2 eggs, 24 grams with 3 eggs), high fat (approximately 20 grams), very low carbohydrate (approximately 6 grams). This is a protein and fat-focused snack ideal for low-carb needs.

Blood Sugar Impact: Minimal to none. Eggs provide protein and fat with virtually no carbohydrates. Avocado provides healthy fats and fiber. This snack has negligible blood sugar impact and provides excellent satiety for 2 to 3 hours.

Best Use Case: Excellent as a mid-morning or mid-afternoon snack when you need sustained energy without carbohydrates. Ideal for rest days or before Zone 2 cardio when you want fuel without spiking blood sugar. Also works as a quick, portable breakfast. The combination of protein and fat provides lasting satiety and prevents blood sugar crashes.

Substitutions:

- Use soft-boiled or poached eggs instead of hard-boiled for variety.

- Replace avocado with hummus or cottage cheese for different fat/protein profiles.

- Add smoked salmon for additional protein and omega-3s.

- Use different seasonings: za'atar, furikake, or simply salt and pepper.

- Add microgreens or arugula for additional nutrients and volume.

Storage & Meal Prep Tips: Hard-boil a dozen eggs at the beginning of the week and store unpeeled in the refrigerator for up to 5 days. Peel eggs when ready to eat. Slice avocado fresh each time, as it browns quickly. If you must prepare avocado in advance, squeeze lemon or lime juice over it and store in an airtight container for up to 24 hours. This snack takes 2 minutes to assemble with prep done, making it ideal for busy schedules.

Recipe 3: Greek Yogurt Protein Parfait

Prep Time: 5 minutes
Cook Time: 0 minutes
Servings: 1

Ingredients:

- 1 cup plain Greek yogurt (full-fat or 2%)
- 1 scoop vanilla protein powder (optional, for higher protein)
- ¼ cup granola (look for low-sugar versions)
- ½ cup mixed berries (fresh or thawed from frozen)
- 1 tablespoon slivered almonds
- 1 teaspoon chia seeds
- ½ teaspoon cinnamon
- Optional: 1 teaspoon honey or a few drops of stevia

Instructions:

1. In a small bowl, mix Greek yogurt with protein powder if using until smooth.
2. In a glass, jar, or bowl, layer half the yogurt mixture.
3. Add half the berries, half the granola, and half the almonds.
4. Repeat layers with remaining yogurt, berries, granola, and almonds.
5. Top with chia seeds and a dusting of cinnamon.
6. Drizzle with optional honey if desired.
7. Eat immediately or refrigerate for up to 2 hours.

Macronutrient Focus: High protein (approximately 30 grams without protein powder, 50+ grams with), moderate fat (approximately 12 grams), moderate carbohydrate (approximately 38 grams). This is a balanced snack or recovery meal.

Blood Sugar Impact: Low to moderate. Greek yogurt is high in protein, which blunts blood sugar response. Berries are among the lowest-glycemic fruits due to fiber content. The moderate amount of granola adds carbohydrates but remains balanced within this high-protein snack. Provides sustained energy without crashes.

Best Use Case: Excellent as a post-workout recovery snack after strength training or moderate cardio. The protein supports muscle recovery, and the carbohydrates from berries and granola help replenish glycogen. Also works as a substantial mid-afternoon snack when you need to bridge the gap between lunch and dinner, or as a quick breakfast. The high protein keeps you satisfied for 3 to 4 hours.

Substitutions:

- Use cottage cheese instead of Greek yogurt for different texture and slightly higher protein.

- Replace granola with toasted oats, crushed whole grain cereal, or omit for lower carbohydrates.

- Use any fruit: diced apple, banana slices, mango, or peaches.

- Add hemp seeds, pumpkin seeds, or walnuts instead of almonds.

- Use ground flaxseed instead of chia seeds.

- Add a tablespoon of nut butter for additional healthy fats and flavor.

Storage & Meal Prep Tips: Greek yogurt parfaits can be assembled up to 24 hours in advance if you layer strategically. Place yogurt in the bottom of a jar, add chia seeds or protein powder mixed in. Add a layer of berries, then granola on top (this prevents it from getting soggy). Store in the refrigerator. The granola will soften slightly but remains acceptable. For best texture, add granola just before eating. Prep multiple jars on Sunday for grab-and-go snacks throughout the week.

Recipe 4: Protein Energy Balls

Prep Time: 15 minutes
Cook Time: 0 minutes
Servings: 12 balls (serving size: 2 balls)

Ingredients:

- 1 cup rolled oats

- ½ cup vanilla or chocolate protein powder

- ½ cup natural almond butter or peanut butter

- ¼ cup honey or maple syrup

- ¼ cup ground flaxseed

- ¼ cup mini dark chocolate chips (70% or higher)

- 2 tablespoons chia seeds

- 1 teaspoon vanilla extract

- Pinch of salt

- 2-3 tablespoons water or almond milk (if needed for binding)

Instructions:

1. In a large bowl, combine rolled oats, protein powder, ground flaxseed, chia seeds, and salt.

2. Add almond butter, honey, and vanilla extract. Mix thoroughly with a spatula or your hands until well combined.

3. Fold in dark chocolate chips.

4. If mixture is too dry and won't hold together, add water or almond milk 1 tablespoon at a time until mixture is sticky and moldable.

5. Using your hands, roll mixture into 12 balls, approximately 1.5 inches in diameter. Pack firmly so they hold together.

6. Place balls on a plate or baking sheet lined with parchment paper.

7. Refrigerate for at least 30 minutes to firm up before eating.

Macronutrient Focus: High protein (approximately 10 grams per 2 balls), moderate fat (approximately 12 grams), moderate carbohydrate (approximately 24 grams). These are balanced, portable energy.

Blood Sugar Impact: Low to moderate. Oats provide complex carbohydrates with fiber. The protein powder and nut butter add significant protein and fat that slow glucose absorption. Honey adds some simple sugars, but the overall blood sugar response remains moderate due to the protein, fat, and fiber content. Provides sustained energy for 2 to 3 hours.

Best Use Case: Excellent as a pre-workout snack 30 to 60 minutes before training when you need easily digestible fuel. Also works as a mid-afternoon snack to prevent excessive hunger before dinner, or as a portable option when traveling. The combination of protein, healthy fats, and carbohydrates makes these versatile for various situations. Not ideal immediately post-workout, as the fat slows digestion.

Substitutions:

- Replace oats with quinoa flakes or puffed rice cereal for different texture.

- Use sunflower seed butter or cashew butter instead of almond butter.

- Replace chocolate chips with dried cranberries, raisins, or chopped dates.

- Add shredded coconut, chopped nuts, or cacao nibs for variety.

- Use cocoa powder instead of chocolate chips for less sugar.

- Replace honey with dates blended into a paste for whole food sweetness.

Storage & Meal Prep Tips: Energy balls are ideal for meal prep. Store in an airtight container in the refrigerator for up to 2 weeks or freeze for up to 3 months. They're portable, require no reheating, and can be eaten anywhere. Pack them in small containers or bags to take to work, the gym, or while traveling. Let frozen balls thaw for 10 minutes before eating, or eat them semi-frozen for a firmer texture. Make a double batch and freeze half for later.

Recipe 5: Turkey and Cheese Roll-Ups

Prep Time: 5 minutes
Cook Time: 0 minutes
Servings: 1

Ingredients:

- 4 slices deli turkey breast (look for nitrate-free, minimally processed)

- 2 slices cheese (cheddar, Swiss, or provolone)

- 2 tablespoons hummus or cream cheese

- ¼ avocado, sliced thin

- 4-6 cucumber spears or bell pepper strips

- Fresh spinach or arugula leaves

- Dijon mustard or hot sauce (optional)

Instructions:

1. Lay turkey slices flat on a clean surface or cutting board.

2. Spread a thin layer of hummus or cream cheese on each turkey slice.

3. Add a few spinach or arugula leaves to each slice.

4. Cut cheese slices in half and place one half on each turkey slice.

5. Add avocado slices and cucumber or bell pepper strips.

6. Add a small amount of Dijon mustard or hot sauce if desired.

7. Roll each turkey slice tightly from one end to the other, creating a compact roll-up.

8. Secure with toothpicks if needed.

9. Eat immediately or pack for a portable snack.

Macronutrient Focus: High protein (approximately 24 grams), moderate fat (approximately 16 grams), low carbohydrate (approximately 6 grams). This is a protein and fat-focused snack ideal for low-carb needs.

Blood Sugar Impact: Minimal. Turkey provides lean protein with no carbohydrates. Cheese and avocado provide fat. Vegetables provide fiber and minimal carbohydrates. This snack has negligible blood sugar impact and provides excellent satiety.

Best Use Case: Excellent as a mid-morning or mid-afternoon snack when you need protein without carbohydrates. Ideal for rest days or before light activity. Also works as a quick, portable lunch option when paired with additional vegetables or fruit. The high protein prevents hunger without interfering with blood sugar or requiring digestion time before activity.

Substitutions:

- Replace turkey with ham, roast beef, or smoked salmon.

- Use dairy-free cheese or omit cheese entirely.

- Replace hummus with avocado, pesto, or mustard.

- Add pickles, olives, or roasted red peppers for additional flavor.

- Use lettuce leaves as wraps instead of turkey for additional vegetables.

- Add sprouts or shredded carrots for crunch.

Storage & Meal Prep Tips: These roll-ups are best assembled fresh, but you can prep components in advance. Pre-slice cheese, cucumbers, and avocado (store avocado with lemon juice to prevent browning). Store in separate containers. Assemble roll-ups each morning or the night before. If assembling ahead, wrap tightly in plastic wrap and refrigerate for up to 24 hours. Remove toothpicks before eating if you used them. Pack with an ice pack if taking to work or traveling.

Recipe 6: Apple Slices with Almond Butter and Cinnamon

Prep Time: 3 minutes
Cook Time: 0 minutes
Servings: 1

Ingredients:

- 1 medium apple (any variety), cored and sliced

- 2 tablespoons natural almond butter (or peanut butter)

- ½ teaspoon cinnamon

- Optional: 1 tablespoon hemp seeds or chia seeds

- Optional: a few dark chocolate chips (70% or higher)

Instructions:

1. Core and slice apple into wedges (approximately 8-10 slices).

2. Arrange apple slices on a plate.

3. Place almond butter in a small bowl for dipping, or spread thinly on each apple slice.

4. Sprinkle cinnamon over apple slices and almond butter.

5. Sprinkle with optional hemp seeds or chia seeds for additional nutrients.

6. Add a few optional dark chocolate chips for a treat.

7. Eat immediately.

Macronutrient Focus: Moderate protein (approximately 8 grams), moderate fat (approximately 16 grams), moderate carbohydrate (approximately 30 grams). This is a balanced snack with carbohydrates from fruit and protein/fat from nut butter.

Blood Sugar Impact: Moderate. Apples contain natural sugars but also significant fiber, especially if you eat the skin. The almond butter provides protein and healthy fats that slow the absorption of carbohydrates from the apple. Cinnamon may help improve insulin sensitivity. The overall blood sugar response is moderate and appropriate for a snack.

Best Use Case: Excellent as a pre-workout snack 45 to 90 minutes before training. The carbohydrates from the apple provide readily available energy, while the fat from almond butter provides sustained fuel. Also works as a mid-afternoon snack when you need energy and satiety. The natural sweetness satisfies cravings without processed sugar. Good for both training and rest days.

Substitutions:

- Use pear, banana, or strawberries instead of apple.

- Replace almond butter with peanut butter, cashew butter, or sunflower seed butter.

- Use honey or maple syrup drizzled over apple for additional sweetness (though not necessary).

- Add a sprinkle of sea salt for sweet-salty contrast.

- Use sliced apple with cottage cheese for higher protein and lower fat.

Storage & Meal Prep Tips: This snack is best assembled fresh, as apple slices brown when exposed to air. If you must prep in advance, toss apple slices with lemon juice to prevent browning and store in an airtight container in the refrigerator for up to 24 hours. Pack almond butter separately in a small container. Assemble just before eating. You can also pre-portion almond butter into small containers at the beginning of the week for grab-and-go convenience.

Recipe 7: Cottage Cheese Power Bowl

Prep Time: 5 minutes
Cook Time: 0 minutes
Servings: 1

Ingredients:

- 1 cup cottage cheese (full-fat or low-fat)
- ¼ cup cherry tomatoes, halved
- ¼ cup cucumber, diced
- 2 tablespoons pumpkin seeds or sunflower seeds
- 1 tablespoon hemp seeds
- 1 tablespoon olive oil
- 1 teaspoon everything bagel seasoning
- Fresh dill or basil, chopped
- Salt and black pepper to taste
- Optional: a few olives or avocado slices

Instructions:

1. Place cottage cheese in a bowl.
2. Top with cherry tomatoes and cucumber.
3. Sprinkle with pumpkin seeds and hemp seeds.
4. Drizzle with olive oil.
5. Season with everything bagel seasoning, fresh herbs, salt, and pepper.
6. Add optional olives or avocado slices.
7. Mix together or eat in layers.

Macronutrient Focus: High protein (approximately 28 grams), moderate fat (approximately 18 grams), low carbohydrate (approximately 10 grams). This is a protein and fat-focused savory snack.

Blood Sugar Impact: Minimal. Cottage cheese provides high protein with minimal carbohydrates. Vegetables provide fiber and minimal carbohydrates. Healthy fats from olive oil and seeds slow any blood sugar response. This snack has very low blood sugar impact and provides excellent satiety.

Best Use Case: Excellent as a substantial mid-afternoon snack when you need protein and satiety without carbohydrates. Ideal for rest days or before/after Zone 2 cardio. Also works as a quick, high-protein breakfast or light lunch. The savory profile makes this satisfying without triggering sugar cravings. Keeps you full for 3 to 4 hours.

Substitutions:

- Use Greek yogurt instead of cottage cheese for different texture.
- Make it sweet instead: use berries, honey, cinnamon, and nuts instead of savory ingredients.

- Add cooked quinoa or chickpeas for additional carbohydrates and fiber.

- Use different vegetables: bell peppers, radishes, or carrots.

- Replace seeds with chopped nuts: almonds, walnuts, or pistachios.

- Add smoked salmon or hard-boiled egg for additional protein.

Storage & Meal Prep Tips: This bowl is best assembled fresh, but you can prep components in advance. Pre-chop vegetables and store in containers. Pre-portion cottage cheese into individual containers. Keep toppings separate until ready to eat. Assembled bowls can be stored in the refrigerator for up to 24 hours, but vegetables may release water and make the cottage cheese watery. For best texture, assemble just before eating.

Recipe 8: Protein Banana Oat Muffins

Prep Time: 10 minutes
Cook Time: 18 minutes
Servings: 12 muffins (serving size: 1-2 muffins)

Ingredients:

- 2 cups rolled oats

- 2 ripe bananas, mashed

- 2 large eggs

- ½ cup vanilla protein powder

- ½ cup unsweetened applesauce

- ¼ cup honey or maple syrup

- ¼ cup almond milk or milk of choice

- 1 teaspoon baking powder

- 1 teaspoon baking soda

- 1 teaspoon cinnamon

- 1 teaspoon vanilla extract

- Pinch of salt

- Optional: ½ cup dark chocolate chips, blueberries, or chopped walnuts

Instructions:

1. Preheat oven to 350°F (175°C). Line a 12-cup muffin tin with paper liners or grease with cooking spray.

2. In a blender or food processor, blend rolled oats until they form a flour-like consistency (or use oat flour).

3. In a large bowl, mash bananas with a fork until smooth.

4. Add eggs, applesauce, honey, almond milk, and vanilla extract to the mashed bananas. Whisk until well combined.

5. In a separate bowl, combine oat flour, protein powder, baking powder, baking soda, cinnamon, and salt.

6. Add dry ingredients to wet ingredients and stir until just combined. Don't overmix.

7. Fold in optional chocolate chips, blueberries, or walnuts if using.

8. Divide batter evenly among 12 muffin cups, filling each about 2/3 full.

9. Bake for 16 to 18 minutes until a toothpick inserted in the center comes out clean and tops are lightly golden.

10. Remove from oven and let cool in the pan for 5 minutes, then transfer to a wire rack to cool completely.

Macronutrient Focus: High protein (approximately 8 grams per muffin), moderate fat (approximately 4 grams), moderate carbohydrate (approximately 22 grams). These are balanced, portable, and satisfying.

Blood Sugar Impact: Low to moderate. Oats provide complex carbohydrates with fiber. Bananas add natural sweetness and carbohydrates. The protein powder adds significant protein that slows glucose absorption. Applesauce reduces the need for added sugar. The overall blood sugar response is moderate and appropriate for a pre-workout snack or recovery meal.

Best Use Case: Excellent as a pre-workout snack 60 to 90 minutes before training. The carbohydrates provide readily available energy while the protein prevents hunger. Also works as a post-workout recovery snack when paired with additional protein, or as a portable breakfast option. These muffins are versatile and can be eaten on training or rest days depending on portion size.

Substitutions:

- Replace bananas with ½ cup pumpkin puree or mashed sweet potato.

- Use any protein powder flavor: vanilla, chocolate, or unflavored.

- Replace honey with mashed dates or additional banana for whole food sweetness.

- Add shredded carrots or zucchini for additional vegetables (squeeze out excess moisture).

- Use different mix-ins: dried cranberries, coconut flakes, or cacao nibs.

- Make them lower-carb by reducing oats to 1½ cups and adding ½ cup almond flour.

Storage & Meal Prep Tips: These muffins are ideal for meal prep. Let cool completely and store in an airtight container at room temperature for up to 3 days or in the refrigerator for up to 5 days. They also freeze beautifully for up to 3 months. Freeze individually wrapped in plastic wrap, then place in a freezer bag. Thaw at room temperature for 1 hour or microwave for 20 to 30 seconds. Make a double batch on Sunday to have grab-and-go snacks throughout the week.

Recipe 9: Tuna Salad on Cucumber Rounds

Prep Time: 10 minutes
Cook Time: 0 minutes
Servings: 2

Ingredients:

- 2 cans (5 ounces each) tuna in water, drained

- 2 tablespoons Greek yogurt or mayonnaise

- 1 celery stalk, finely diced

- 2 tablespoons red onion, finely diced

- 1 tablespoon fresh dill, chopped (or 1 teaspoon dried)

- 1 teaspoon Dijon mustard

- 1 teaspoon lemon juice

- Salt and black pepper to taste

- 2 large cucumbers, sliced into ½-inch rounds (approximately 20-24 rounds)

- Optional: everything bagel seasoning or paprika for garnish

Instructions:

1. In a medium bowl, combine drained tuna, Greek yogurt or mayonnaise, diced celery, red onion, dill, Dijon mustard, and lemon juice.

2. Mix well until combined. Season with salt and pepper to taste.

3. Slice cucumbers into ½-inch thick rounds. Pat dry with paper towels if they're very watery.

4. Arrange cucumber rounds on a plate or platter.

5. Top each cucumber round with approximately 1 tablespoon of tuna salad.

6. Garnish with optional everything bagel seasoning or paprika.

7. Serve immediately or refrigerate for up to 2 hours before serving.

Macronutrient Focus: High protein (approximately 32 grams per serving), low fat (approximately 4 grams with Greek yogurt, 12 grams with mayonnaise), very low carbohydrate (approximately 6 grams). This is a lean, protein-focused snack.

Blood Sugar Impact: Minimal to none. Tuna provides lean protein with no carbohydrates. Cucumbers provide volume, crunch, and hydration with minimal carbohydrates. This snack has negligible blood sugar impact and provides excellent satiety.

Best Use Case: Excellent as a mid-afternoon snack when you need protein without carbohydrates or fat. Ideal for rest days or before/after Zone 2 cardio. Also works as an appetizer or light lunch. The omega-3s from tuna (especially if using albacore) support recovery and reduce inflammation. The high protein content keeps you satisfied for 2 to 3 hours.

Substitutions:

- Replace tuna with canned salmon, chicken, or cooked shrimp.

- Use celery sticks, bell pepper boats, or endive leaves instead of cucumber rounds.

- Replace Greek yogurt with avocado mashed into the tuna for healthy fats.

- Add capers, pickles, or olives for additional flavor.

- Use fresh parsley or cilantro instead of dill.

- Serve on whole grain crackers or rice cakes for additional carbohydrates.

Storage & Meal Prep Tips: Tuna salad can be made up to 3 days in advance and stored in an airtight container in the refrigerator. Slice cucumbers fresh each day to prevent them from becoming watery and soggy. If you must slice in advance, store in a container lined with paper towels to absorb excess moisture. Assemble cucumber rounds with tuna salad just before eating or serving. This is a quick, protein-rich option that takes minutes to prepare with prepped components.

Recipe 10: Sweet Potato and Protein Pancakes (Recovery Version)

Prep Time: 5 minutes
Cook Time: 10 minutes
Servings: 2 (approximately 6 small pancakes)

Ingredients:

- ½ cup cooked sweet potato, mashed (about 1 small sweet potato)

- 2 large eggs

- 1 scoop vanilla protein powder

- 2 tablespoons oat flour or almond flour

- ½ teaspoon baking powder

- ½ teaspoon cinnamon

- ¼ teaspoon vanilla extract

- Pinch of salt

- Coconut oil or butter for cooking

For Topping:

- 2 tablespoons almond butter or peanut butter

- ½ banana, sliced

- Optional: maple syrup or honey

Instructions:

1. In a medium bowl, combine mashed sweet potato, eggs, protein powder, oat flour, baking powder, cinnamon, vanilla extract, and salt. Whisk until smooth. The batter will be thick.

2. Heat a non-stick skillet or griddle over medium-low heat. Add a small amount of coconut oil or butter.

3. Pour approximately ¼ cup of batter per pancake onto the skillet. Use the back of a spoon to gently spread into a circle.

4. Cook for 2 to 3 minutes until bubbles form on the surface and edges begin to set.

5. Flip carefully and cook for another 2 minutes until golden brown and cooked through.

6. Repeat with remaining batter, adding more oil as needed.

7. Serve warm topped with almond butter, banana slices, and optional maple syrup or honey.

Macronutrient Focus: High protein (approximately 25 grams per serving), moderate fat (approximately 14 grams), moderate to high carbohydrate (approximately 40 grams). This is a complete recovery meal with balanced macronutrients.

Blood Sugar Impact: Moderate. Sweet potatoes provide complex carbohydrates with fiber. The protein powder and eggs add significant protein that slows glucose absorption. The overall blood sugar response is moderate and appropriate for post-workout recovery. Provides sustained energy and supports muscle recovery.

Best Use Case: Excellent as a post-workout recovery meal within 60 to 90 minutes after strength training or high-intensity cardio. The combination of protein and carbohydrates supports muscle protein synthesis and glycogen replenishment. Also works as a substantial pre-workout meal 2 to 3 hours before training, or as a satisfying breakfast on training days. The sweet potato provides quality carbohydrates that fuel performance and recovery.

Substitutions:

- Replace sweet potato with mashed banana or pumpkin puree.

- Use any protein powder flavor: vanilla, chocolate, or unflavored.

- Replace oat flour with whole wheat flour or additional almond flour.

- Top with Greek yogurt instead of nut butter for additional protein.

- Add blueberries or chocolate chips to the batter for variety.

- Use different nut butters: cashew butter or sunflower seed butter.

Storage & Meal Prep Tips: These pancakes can be made ahead and stored in the refrigerator for up to 4 days or frozen for up to 2 months. Let pancakes cool completely, then layer between sheets of parchment paper and store in an airtight container or freezer bag. Reheat in a toaster, toaster oven, or microwave. Frozen pancakes can be reheated directly from the freezer. Make a large batch on Sunday to have quick post-workout recovery meals throughout the week. Store toppings separately and add fresh when ready to eat.

These ten snack and recovery meal recipes provide strategic nutrition tools to support your training, manage hunger between meals, and optimize recovery. Each recipe serves a specific purpose, whether it's pre-workout fuel, post-workout recovery, or sustained energy between meals.

Notice the distinction between these recipes and typical snack foods. These are not engineered to be hyper-palatable and irresistible. They are not designed to be eaten mindlessly. They are built around whole foods, prioritize protein, and serve a functional purpose in your nutrition plan.

The key to using snacks appropriately is awareness. Ask yourself: am I genuinely hungry, or am I eating out of boredom, stress, or habit? Do I need fuel for training, or am I adequately nourished from my meals? Is this snack supporting my goals, or is it undermining them?

Strategic snacking guidelines:

- Snack when genuinely hungry between meals, not out of habit or boredom

- Use recovery meals within 60 to 90 minutes after intense training

- Choose pre-workout snacks 30 to 90 minutes before training based on digestion needs

- Prioritize protein in all snacks to support satiety and muscle maintenance

- Match carbohydrate content to activity level and timing

- Skip snacking entirely if meals are substantial and spaced appropriately

Remember that the need for snacks varies individually. Some people do well with three substantial meals and no snacks. Others benefit from smaller meals supplemented with strategic snacks. Your training schedule, body size, metabolic health, and daily activity level all influence your needs.

Pay attention to patterns. If you find yourself needing snacks every day at the same time, your meals may be inadequate. If you're snacking out of boredom or stress, address the underlying issue rather than using food as a coping mechanism. If you're genuinely hungry between meals despite eating substantial food, you may need to increase meal size or adjust macronutrient ratios.

Snacking is a tool, not a requirement. Use it strategically, not habitually. When you do snack, make it count with options that support your longevity goals rather than undermining them.

CHAPTER 11: LONGEVITY DRINKS & SIMPLE DESSERTS

Most beverages and desserts sold today are engineered to deliver maximum sugar with minimal nutrition. A single flavored coffee drink can contain 50 grams of sugar. A typical dessert at a restaurant can exceed 80 grams. These are not foods. They are metabolic sabotage dressed up as treats.

But desserts and drinks don't have to undermine your health. When built around whole foods and consumed mindfully, they can satisfy cravings, provide enjoyment, and even contribute nutrients. The key is shifting from sugar-delivery systems to real food that happens to taste good.

This chapter provides five longevity-friendly drinks and five simple desserts. None contain artificial sweeteners or excessive added sugars. All use whole food ingredients. They satisfy without triggering the blood sugar rollercoaster that drives cravings and metabolic dysfunction.

Use these strategically, not habitually. They are occasional additions, not daily requirements.

Recipe 1: Golden Turmeric Latte

Prep Time: 5 minutes
Cook Time: 5 minutes
Servings: 1

Ingredients:

- 1 cup unsweetened almond milk or milk of choice

- 1 teaspoon turmeric powder

- ½ teaspoon cinnamon

- ¼ teaspoon ginger powder

- Pinch of black pepper (enhances turmeric absorption)

- 1 teaspoon honey or maple syrup (optional)

- ½ teaspoon vanilla extract

- Optional: ½ teaspoon coconut oil

Instructions:

1. Heat milk in a small saucepan over medium heat until steaming but not boiling.

2. Add turmeric, cinnamon, ginger, black pepper, and optional coconut oil. Whisk continuously for 2 minutes.

3. Remove from heat and stir in vanilla extract and optional honey.

4. Pour into a mug and enjoy warm.

Macronutrient Focus: Minimal macros (approximately 2g protein, 4g fat, 8g carbs with sweetener). This is a functional beverage focused on anti-inflammatory compounds rather than macronutrients.

Blood Sugar Impact: Minimal. The small amount of honey creates negligible blood sugar response. Turmeric and cinnamon may actually improve insulin sensitivity.

Best Use Case: Excellent as an evening drink to reduce inflammation and support recovery. Also works as a warm, soothing beverage any time. The anti-inflammatory properties support joint health and recovery from training.

Storage & Meal Prep Tips: Make a spice blend in advance: combine 4 tablespoons turmeric, 2 tablespoons cinnamon, 1 tablespoon ginger, and 1 teaspoon black pepper. Store in a jar and use 1 teaspoon per serving. The prepared latte is best consumed immediately.

Recipe 2: Green Recovery Smoothie

Prep Time: 5 minutes
Cook Time: 0 minutes
Servings: 1

Ingredients:

- 1 cup fresh spinach
- ½ cup frozen pineapple
- ½ frozen banana
- ½ cup coconut water
- ½ cup unsweetened almond milk
- 1 tablespoon chia seeds
- Juice of ½ lime
- Optional: small piece of fresh ginger

Instructions:

1. Add all ingredients to a blender.
2. Blend until smooth, about 60 seconds.
3. Add more liquid if too thick.
4. Drink immediately.

Macronutrient Focus: Low protein (4g), minimal fat (5g), moderate carbs (32g). This is a hydrating, micronutrient-rich beverage.

Blood Sugar Impact: Moderate. The fruit provides natural sugars, but fiber from spinach, chia seeds, and fruit slows absorption. Best consumed post-workout when insulin sensitivity is elevated.

Best Use Case: Post-Zone 2 cardio or as a hydrating recovery drink. The coconut water provides electrolytes. Not ideal for heavy strength training due to low protein content.

Recipe 3: Bone Broth with Herbs

Prep Time: 5 minutes
Cook Time: 5 minutes
Servings: 1

Ingredients:

- 1½ cups bone broth (chicken, beef, or fish)

- 1 garlic clove, minced

- ½ teaspoon fresh ginger, grated

- Fresh herbs (parsley, cilantro, or thyme)

- ½ teaspoon apple cider vinegar

- Salt and black pepper to taste

- Optional: red pepper flakes

Instructions:

1. Heat bone broth in a small pot over medium heat.

2. Add garlic and ginger. Simmer for 3 to 4 minutes.

3. Remove from heat. Stir in apple cider vinegar and fresh herbs.

4. Season with salt, pepper, and optional red pepper flakes.

5. Serve hot in a mug.

Macronutrient Focus: High protein (10g), minimal fat (2g), minimal carbs (2g). Rich in collagen and minerals.

Blood Sugar Impact: None. This is pure protein and minerals with no carbohydrates.

Best Use Case: Excellent for recovery, joint health, and gut healing. Drink between meals or before bed. The collagen supports connective tissue repair.

Storage & Meal Prep Tips: Make or buy bone broth in bulk. Store in the refrigerator for up to 5 days or freeze in portions. Reheat and add fresh herbs each time.

Recipe 4: Iced Matcha Latte

Prep Time: 3 minutes
Cook Time: 0 minutes
Servings: 1

Ingredients:

- 1 teaspoon matcha powder

- 2 tablespoons hot water

- 1 cup unsweetened almond milk or milk of choice

- Ice cubes

- Optional: 1 teaspoon honey or a few drops stevia

Instructions:

1. In a small bowl, whisk matcha powder with hot water until smooth and no clumps remain.

2. Fill a glass with ice.

3. Pour milk over ice.

4. Add matcha mixture and stir well.

5. Add optional sweetener if desired.

Macronutrient Focus: Minimal macros (2g protein, 3g fat, 4g carbs). This is a functional beverage providing antioxidants and gentle caffeine.

Blood Sugar Impact: Minimal. Contains virtually no carbohydrates unless sweetened.

Best Use Case: Morning or pre-workout energy boost. Matcha provides sustained energy without the crash of coffee. The L-theanine promotes calm focus.

Recipe 5: Homemade Electrolyte Drink

Prep Time: 3 minutes
Cook Time: 0 minutes
Servings: 1

Ingredients:

- 2 cups water

- Juice of 1 lemon or lime

- ¼ teaspoon sea salt

- 1 tablespoon honey or maple syrup

- Optional: pinch of magnesium powder

Instructions:

1. Combine all ingredients in a large glass or bottle.

2. Shake or stir until dissolved.

3. Drink during or after training.

Macronutrient Focus: Minimal protein/fat, moderate carbs (18g from honey). Provides sodium and electrolytes.

Blood Sugar Impact: Low to moderate. The honey provides some sugar, but it's diluted and consumed during activity when insulin sensitivity is high.

Best Use Case: During or after training sessions longer than 60 minutes, especially in hot weather. Replenishes electrolytes lost through sweat.

Recipe 6: Dark Chocolate Avocado Mousse

Prep Time: 10 minutes (plus 1 hour chilling)
Cook Time: 0 minutes
Servings: 4

Ingredients:

- 2 ripe avocados

- ¼ cup unsweetened cocoa powder

- ¼ cup maple syrup or honey

- ¼ cup unsweetened almond milk

- 1 teaspoon vanilla extract

- Pinch of salt

- Optional: fresh berries and whipped coconut cream for topping

Instructions:

1. Add all ingredients to a food processor or blender.

2. Blend until completely smooth and creamy, scraping down sides as needed.

3. Taste and adjust sweetness if needed.

4. Divide into four small bowls or ramekins.

5. Refrigerate for at least 1 hour to set.

6. Top with optional berries and coconut cream before serving.

Macronutrient Focus: Moderate fat (15g), low protein (3g), moderate carbs (22g). The avocado provides healthy fats and creates rich, creamy texture.

Blood Sugar Impact: Low to moderate. The fat from avocado and fiber slow the absorption of sugars from maple syrup and cocoa. This is a satisfying dessert that won't spike blood sugar.

Best Use Case: Occasional dessert when you want something sweet and satisfying. The healthy fats provide satiety. Dark chocolate and avocado both contain beneficial compounds.

Storage & Meal Prep Tips: Store covered in the refrigerator for up to 3 days. Press plastic wrap directly onto the surface to prevent browning.

Recipe 7: Baked Cinnamon Apples

Prep Time: 5 minutes
Cook Time: 25 minutes
Servings: 2

Ingredients:

- 2 large apples, cored and sliced

- 1 tablespoon coconut oil, melted

- 1 teaspoon cinnamon

- ¼ teaspoon nutmeg

- 1 tablespoon chopped walnuts or pecans

- Optional: 1 teaspoon honey and Greek yogurt for serving

Instructions:

1. Preheat oven to 375°F (190°C).

2. Arrange apple slices in a baking dish.

3. Drizzle with melted coconut oil.

4. Sprinkle with cinnamon and nutmeg.

5. Top with chopped nuts.

6. Bake for 20 to 25 minutes until apples are tender.

7. Serve warm with optional honey drizzle and Greek yogurt.

Macronutrient Focus: Low protein (2g), moderate fat (10g), moderate carbs (28g). This is a fruit-based dessert with healthy fats from nuts.

Blood Sugar Impact: Moderate. Apples contain natural sugars and fiber. The coconut oil and nuts slow absorption. Cinnamon may improve insulin sensitivity.

Best Use Case: Occasional dessert on training days when you have room for carbohydrates. The warm, comforting preparation satisfies without processed sugar.

Recipe 8: Protein Chocolate Bark

Prep Time: 10 minutes (plus 1 hour freezing)
Cook Time: 3 minutes
Servings: 12 pieces

Ingredients:

- 8 ounces dark chocolate (70% or higher), chopped

- 2 scoops chocolate protein powder

- ¼ cup almonds, roughly chopped

- 2 tablespoons chia seeds

- 2 tablespoons unsweetened coconut flakes

- Pinch of sea salt

Instructions:

1. Line a baking sheet with parchment paper.

2. Melt chocolate in a double boiler or microwave in 30-second intervals, stirring between each.

3. Once melted, stir in protein powder until smooth.

4. Pour onto prepared baking sheet and spread into a thin, even layer.

5. Sprinkle with almonds, chia seeds, and coconut flakes.

6. Finish with a light sprinkle of sea salt.

7. Freeze for 1 hour until firm.

8. Break into 12 pieces and store in the freezer.

Macronutrient Focus: Moderate protein (6g), moderate fat (9g), low carbs (8g). This is a protein-boosted dessert with healthy fats.

Blood Sugar Impact: Low. Dark chocolate contains minimal sugar. The protein powder, healthy fats, and fiber create stable blood sugar response.

Best Use Case: Occasional sweet treat when you want chocolate. The protein content makes this more satisfying than regular candy. Portion control is essential—eat one piece, not the entire batch.

Storage & Meal Prep Tips: Store in an airtight container in the freezer for up to 2 months. The bark will soften at room temperature, so keep frozen until ready to eat.

Recipe 9: Berry Chia Pudding

Prep Time: 5 minutes (plus 4 hours or overnight setting)
Cook Time: 0 minutes
Servings: 2

Ingredients:

- 1 cup unsweetened almond milk
- ¼ cup chia seeds
- ½ cup mixed berries, mashed
- 1 tablespoon honey or maple syrup
- ½ teaspoon vanilla extract
- Optional: additional fresh berries for topping

Instructions:

1. In a bowl, whisk together almond milk, chia seeds, mashed berries, honey, and vanilla.
2. Divide between two jars or containers.
3. Cover and refrigerate for at least 4 hours or overnight.
4. The chia seeds will absorb liquid and create a pudding-like consistency.
5. Stir before serving and top with fresh berries if desired.

Macronutrient Focus: Moderate protein (6g), moderate fat (9g), moderate carbs (22g). Chia seeds provide protein, omega-3s, and fiber.

Blood Sugar Impact: Low. The fiber and healthy fats from chia seeds slow the absorption of sugars from berries and honey.

Best Use Case: Breakfast or dessert option. The fiber and protein provide satiety. Can be made in advance for grab-and-go convenience.

Recipe 10: Frozen Banana Bites

Prep Time: 10 minutes (plus 2 hours freezing)
Cook Time: 0 minutes
Servings: 12 bites

Ingredients:

- 2 bananas, cut into ½-inch slices

- 2 tablespoons almond butter or peanut butter

- 4 ounces dark chocolate (70% or higher), melted

- 2 tablespoons chopped peanuts or almonds

- Sea salt for sprinkling

Instructions:

1. Line a baking sheet with parchment paper.

2. Spread a small amount of almond butter on half the banana slices.

3. Top with remaining banana slices to create sandwiches.

4. Place on prepared baking sheet and freeze for 1 hour.

5. Once firm, dip each banana bite halfway into melted dark chocolate.

6. Sprinkle with chopped nuts and a pinch of sea salt.

7. Return to freezer for 1 hour until chocolate hardens.

8. Store in the freezer in an airtight container.

Macronutrient Focus: Low protein (3g), moderate fat (7g), moderate carbs (18g). This is a fruit-based treat with healthy fats from nut butter and dark chocolate.

Blood Sugar Impact: Moderate. Bananas contain natural sugars, but the nut butter and dark chocolate provide fat that slows absorption. Best consumed in moderation.

Best Use Case: Occasional dessert when you want something sweet and satisfying. The frozen texture makes these feel indulgent. Portion control is key—one or two bites, not the entire batch.

[CHAPTER INTEGRATION]

These drinks and desserts prove that you don't need processed sugar and artificial ingredients to enjoy satisfying flavors. Each recipe uses whole foods, provides some nutritional value, and satisfies without triggering blood sugar chaos.

But remember: these are occasional additions, not daily staples. Dessert every night creates habituation and undermines metabolic health. Save these for special occasions, post-training treats, or when you genuinely want something sweet—not as automatic daily rituals.

The best dessert is often none at all. When your meals are satisfying and your blood sugar is stable, sweet cravings diminish naturally. You stop needing dessert to feel complete.

Use these recipes strategically. Enjoy them mindfully. And most importantly, don't let desserts and drinks become another source of stress or guilt. Occasional treats are part of a sustainable, lifelong approach to eating.

CHAPTER 12: HOW TO TRAIN FOR DECADES

Most people train as if they're preparing for a competition that will never come. They push hard, ignore pain, skip recovery, and burn out within months. They confuse intensity with effectiveness and suffering with progress.

Longevity training requires a different mindset. It's not about how hard you can push today. It's about how well you can move fifty years from now. It's about building capacity that lasts, not chasing short-term gains that break you down.

This chapter establishes the principles that make sustainable training possible. You'll learn the difference between training minimums and ideals, how to prevent injury before it happens, how to progress without burnout, and when to push versus pull back.

These principles guide the 12-week program that follows. Master them, and you'll train not just for months, but for decades.

Training Minimums vs Ideals

There's a crucial difference between the minimum effective dose of training and the optimal dose. The minimum is what you need to maintain capacity and prevent decline. The ideal is what produces meaningful progress without exceeding recovery capacity.

The Minimum:

- 2 strength training sessions per week

- 90 minutes of Zone 2 cardio per week

- 10 minutes of mobility work most days

This minimum prevents muscle loss, maintains cardiovascular fitness, and preserves joint health. It's enough to keep you functional and healthy. But it won't build significant capacity or drive adaptation.

The Ideal:

- 3-4 strength training sessions per week

- 150-180 minutes of Zone 2 cardio per week

- 1 high-intensity session per week

- Daily mobility work

This ideal builds strength, improves cardiovascular capacity, and creates meaningful adaptation. It's sustainable for most people with proper recovery.

The gap between minimum and ideal is where you operate based on your life circumstances. Busy week? Drop to the minimum. Stress is high? Pull back. Recovered and energized? Push toward the ideal.

Flexibility prevents the all-or-nothing thinking that destroys consistency. Some training is always better than no training. Don't abandon the minimum because you can't achieve the ideal.

Injury Prevention Mindset

Injuries don't happen randomly. They're the result of accumulated stress, poor movement patterns, inadequate recovery, or ignoring warning signs. Prevention requires vigilance and humility.

Move Well Before Moving Heavy

Technique matters more than load. Lifting heavy weight with poor form creates joint stress and injury risk that accumulates over time. Master movement patterns with lighter loads before adding weight.

Every rep should look like your best rep. When technique degrades, the set is over. Ego lifting has no place in longevity training.

Respect Pain Signals

Discomfort from effort is normal. Sharp pain, joint pain, or pain that worsens during a set is a warning. Stop immediately. Pushing through pain creates injuries that take months to heal and interrupt training far longer than one missed workout.

Learn the difference between muscle fatigue and joint stress. The first is productive. The second is destructive.

Progressive Loading

Add weight gradually. A good rule: increase load by 5-10% only after you can complete all prescribed sets and reps with good form. Rushing progress leads to breakdown.

Strength builds slowly. Tendons and ligaments adapt even slower. Patience prevents injury.

Joint-Friendly Exercise Selection

Some exercises are higher risk for certain individuals. If an exercise consistently causes pain despite good form, replace it. There are always alternatives.

Barbell back squats bothering your knees? Try goblet squats, split squats, or leg press. Bench press irritating your shoulders? Try dumbbell presses, push-ups, or landmine presses.

The best exercise is the one you can do pain-free with good form.

Progression Without Burnout

Progress requires stress. But too much stress without adequate recovery creates overtraining, injury, and burnout. The key is calibrating intensity to recovery capacity.

Progressive Overload Strategies

Progress doesn't always mean adding weight. You can progress by:

- Adding reps: 3 sets of 8 becomes 3 sets of 10

- Adding sets: 3 sets becomes 4 sets

- Slowing tempo: 2-second eccentric becomes 4-second eccentric

- Reducing rest periods: 90 seconds becomes 60 seconds

- Improving technique: deeper range of motion, better control

Rotate through these methods to avoid plateaus while managing joint stress.

Deload Weeks

Every 4-6 weeks, take a deload week. Reduce training volume by 40-50% and intensity by 20-30%. This allows your body to recover fully and supercompensate.

A deload week might look like:

- 2 strength sessions instead of 4

- Same exercises, but 2 sets instead of 4

- Lighter weights that feel easy

- Normal Zone 2 cardio but no high-intensity work

Deloads feel like stepping backward. They're actually essential for moving forward. Most people need them more often than they think.

Listening to Your Body

Track subjective markers:

- Sleep quality

- Energy levels

- Mood and motivation

- Persistent soreness

- Performance decline

If multiple markers are off, reduce training volume or take an extra rest day. Pushing through only prolongs recovery time.

When to Push vs Pull Back

Knowing when to train hard and when to ease off separates sustainable training from burnout.

Push When:

- You feel energized and recovered

- Sleep has been good for several nights

- Motivation is high

- Movement feels smooth and controlled

- No lingering soreness or pain

Pull Back When:

- Sleep has been poor for multiple nights

- Stress is unusually high (work, relationships, life events)

- Persistent fatigue that doesn't resolve with rest

- Movement feels sluggish or uncoordinated

- Soreness lingers beyond 48 hours

- Elevated resting heart rate (5-10 bpm above baseline)

- Decreased motivation or feelings of dread about training

Pulling back doesn't mean doing nothing. It means reducing intensity, volume, or both. Light movement aids recovery better than complete rest.

The 80/20 Rule

Approximately 80% of your training should feel sustainable and moderate. Only 20% should feel truly challenging or hard. If every session feels like a battle, you're training too hard too often.

Most people do the opposite: they train moderately hard all the time, never easy enough to recover fully or hard enough to drive adaptation. This creates chronic fatigue without progress.

Train easy when you're supposed to train easy. Train hard when you're supposed to train hard. The discipline is in both directions.

These principles form the foundation of sustainable training. Training minimums provide a baseline during challenging periods. The injury prevention mindset keeps you training for decades rather than months. Progression strategies drive adaptation without burnout. And knowing when to push versus pull back prevents the overtraining that destroys consistency.

The 12-week program in the next chapter applies these principles systematically. But the principles matter more than any single program. Programs change. Principles endure.

Before moving to the program, internalize these concepts:

- Consistency beats intensity

- Some training is always better than no training

- Pain is a warning, not a challenge to overcome

- Progress is measured in years, not weeks

- Recovery is when adaptation happens

Write these down. Return to them when motivation fades or when you're tempted to push beyond your capacity. They will guide you through decades of training, long after this program ends.

Training for longevity is not about being the strongest person in the gym today. It's about being strong enough to live fully at seventy, eighty, and beyond. That requires patience, intelligence, and respect for the process.

The program begins now.

CHAPTER 13: THE 12-WEEK LONGEVITY FITNESS PLAN

This is the roadmap. Twelve weeks of structured training designed to build strength, cardiovascular capacity, mobility, and stability in a way that's sustainable, progressive, and adaptable to your life.

The program is divided into three four-week phases:

Phase 1 (Weeks 1-4): Foundation Establish movement patterns, build work capacity, and create training consistency.

Phase 2 (Weeks 5-8): Capacity Building Increase training volume and intensity while maintaining good form and recovery.

Phase 3 (Weeks 9-12): Integration & Sustainability Optimize performance, test progress, and transition to long-term maintenance.

Each week includes strength training sessions, Zone 2 cardio, mobility work, and optional conditioning. The plan assumes 4-6 training days per week, with sessions lasting 30-75 minutes.

This is a template, not a rigid prescription. Adjust based on your schedule, recovery capacity, and life circumstances. The principles matter more than perfect execution.

Program Overview and Guidelines

Training Frequency:

- Strength Training: 3 sessions per week (can be 2 during busy weeks)

- Zone 2 Cardio: 3 sessions per week, 30-60 minutes each

- Mobility Work: Daily, 5-10 minutes

- Optional Conditioning: 1 session per week

Equipment Needed:

- Basic: Bodyweight, resistance bands, dumbbells

- Ideal: Barbell, squat rack, bench, pull-up bar

- Cardio: Access to walking/running route, bike, rower, or elliptical

Rest Days: At least 1-2 complete rest days per week. Active recovery (light walking, gentle stretching) is encouraged.

Progression Principles:

- Add weight when you can complete all sets with 1-2 reps in reserve

- Increase reps before adding weight if technique needs refinement

- Take deload weeks as prescribed (Week 4, Week 8, Week 12)

Exercise Notation:

- Sets × Reps: Example: 3×8 means 3 sets of 8 reps

- Tempo: Example: 3-1-1-0 means 3-second eccentric, 1-second pause, 1-second concentric, no pause at top

- Rest: Time between sets

Phase 1: Foundation (Weeks 1-4)

Goals:

- Master fundamental movement patterns

- Build aerobic base with Zone 2 cardio

- Establish consistent training rhythm

- Develop body awareness and mobility

Training Structure:

- Strength: 3 sessions per week (Monday, Wednesday, Friday)

- Zone 2: 3 sessions per week (Tuesday, Thursday, Saturday)

- Mobility: Daily, 5-10 minutes

- Rest: Sunday + as needed

Week 1: Movement Foundation

[Strength Training - Day 1: Full Body A]

Warm-Up (10 minutes):

- 5 minutes light cardio (walk, bike, or row)

- Arm circles: 10 each direction

- Leg swings: 10 each direction per leg

- Bodyweight squats: 15 reps

- Push-ups (modified if needed): 10 reps

- Cat-cow stretch: 10 reps

Main Workout:

1. **Goblet Squat**

   o 3 sets × 10 reps

- o Rest: 90 seconds

- o Focus: Depth, upright torso, knees tracking over toes

2. **Dumbbell Romanian Deadlift (RDL)**

- o 3 sets × 10 reps

- o Rest: 90 seconds

- o Focus: Hip hinge pattern, maintain neutral spine

3. **Push-Up (or Incline Push-Up)**

- o 3 sets × 8-12 reps

- o Rest: 60 seconds

- o Focus: Full range of motion, elbows 45 degrees from body

4. **Dumbbell Single-Arm Row**

- o 3 sets × 10 reps per arm

- o Rest: 60 seconds

- o Focus: Pull with elbow, minimize torso rotation

5. **Plank Hold**

- o 3 sets × 20-30 seconds

- o Rest: 60 seconds

- o Focus: Neutral spine, engaged core

6. **Glute Bridge**

- o 3 sets × 15 reps

- o Rest: 45 seconds

- o Focus: Full hip extension, squeeze glutes at top

Cool-Down (5 minutes):

- Child's pose: 60 seconds

- Hamstring stretch: 30 seconds per leg

- Hip flexor stretch: 30 seconds per leg

- Chest stretch: 30 seconds

[Strength Training - Day 2: Full Body B]

Warm-Up (10 minutes):

- Same as Day 1

Main Workout:

1. **Dumbbell Reverse Lunge**

   - 3 sets × 8 reps per leg
   - Rest: 90 seconds
   - Focus: Control, knee alignment, upright torso

2. **Dumbbell Bench Press (or Floor Press)**

   - 3 sets × 10 reps
   - Rest: 90 seconds
   - Focus: Full range of motion, stable shoulder blades

3. **Lat Pulldown (or Assisted Pull-Up)**

   - 3 sets × 10 reps
   - Rest: 90 seconds
   - Focus: Pull to chest, shoulder blades down and back

4. **Dumbbell Shoulder Press**

   - 3 sets × 8 reps
   - Rest: 60 seconds
   - Focus: Press straight overhead, avoid arching back

5. **Pallof Press (or Anti-Rotation Hold)**

   - 3 sets × 10 reps per side
   - Rest: 60 seconds
   - Focus: Resist rotation, maintain stable torso

6. **Dead Bug**

   - 3 sets × 10 reps per side
   - Rest: 45 seconds
   - Focus: Keep lower back pressed to floor

Cool-Down (5 minutes):

- Same as Day 1

[Strength Training - Day 3: Full Body C]

Warm-Up (10 minutes):

- Same as Day 1

Main Workout:

1. **Split Squat (Non-Elevated)**

   - 3 sets × 8 reps per leg
   - Rest: 90 seconds
   - Focus: Balance, front knee alignment

2. **Dumbbell Step-Up**

   - 3 sets × 8 reps per leg
   - Rest: 60 seconds
   - Focus: Drive through front heel, control descent

3. **Dumbbell Row (Two-Arm, Bent Over)**

   - 3 sets × 10 reps
   - Rest: 90 seconds
   - Focus: Hip hinge position, pull elbows back

4. **Landmine Press (or Dumbbell Incline Press)**

   - 3 sets × 10 reps
   - Rest: 60 seconds
   - Focus: Controlled press, stable core

5. **Farmer's Carry**

   - 3 sets × 30-40 seconds
   - Rest: 90 seconds
   - Focus: Upright posture, stable shoulders

6. **Bird Dog**

   - 3 sets × 8 reps per side

- o   Rest: 45 seconds

- o   Focus: Opposite arm and leg, stable spine

Cool-Down (5 minutes):

- •   Same as Day 1

[Zone 2 Cardio Sessions - Week 1]

Format: Choose your preferred modality: walking, jogging, cycling, rowing, swimming, or elliptical.

Intensity: You should be able to hold a conversation but not sing comfortably. Nasal breathing only is a good indicator. Heart rate typically 60-70% of max.

Duration:

- •   Session 1 (Tuesday): 30 minutes

- •   Session 2 (Thursday): 30 minutes

- •   Session 3 (Saturday): 40 minutes

Notes: Stay consistent with intensity. Too easy won't drive adaptation. Too hard exceeds Zone 2 and interferes with strength recovery.

[Daily Mobility Work - Week 1]

Morning or Evening Routine (5-10 minutes):

1. **Cat-Cow Stretch**: 10 slow reps

2. **90/90 Hip Stretch**: 30 seconds per side

3. **Thoracic Rotation**: 8 reps per side

4. **Deep Squat Hold**: 30-60 seconds

5. **Shoulder Pass-Through (with band or towel)**: 10 reps

6. **Ankle Circles**: 10 each direction per foot

Perform this sequence daily, preferably at the same time to build habit.

Week 2: Volume Introduction

Strength Training: Same exercises as Week 1. Increase to 4 sets for main movements (exercises 1-4 in each session). Keep accessory work (exercises 5-6) at 3 sets. Focus on improving technique and control.

Zone 2 Cardio:

- •   Session 1: 35 minutes

- Session 2: 35 minutes

- Session 3: 45 minutes

Mobility: Same routine as Week 1, performed daily.

Week 3: Intensity Introduction

Strength Training: Same exercises. Maintain 4 sets for main movements. Slightly increase weight if Week 2 felt manageable with 1-2 reps in reserve. Focus on controlled eccentric (lowering) phase.

Zone 2 Cardio:

- Session 1: 40 minutes

- Session 2: 40 minutes

- Session 3: 50 minutes

Mobility: Same routine, add 5 minutes of foam rolling before or after training sessions.

Week 4: Deload

Strength Training: Same exercises. Reduce to 2-3 sets per exercise. Reduce weight by 20-30%. Focus entirely on perfect form and feeling good. This is recovery, not testing.

Zone 2 Cardio:

- Session 1: 30 minutes (easy pace)

- Session 2: 30 minutes (easy pace)

- Optional Session 3: 30 minutes or skip entirely

Mobility: Continue daily routine. Add extra stretching or gentle yoga if desired.

Notes: Week 4 is a deload to allow full recovery before Phase 2. You should feel refreshed and ready to push harder by the end of this week.

Phase 2: Capacity Building (Weeks 5-8)

Goals:

- Increase training volume and intensity

- Introduce new movement patterns

- Build work capacity

- Improve cardiovascular fitness with one high-intensity session weekly

Training Structure:

- Strength: 3-4 sessions per week

- Zone 2: 3 sessions per week, 40-60 minutes

- High-Intensity: 1 session per week (Week 6 onward)

- Mobility: Daily

Week 5: Volume Increase

[Strength Training - Day 1: Lower Focus]

Warm-Up (10 minutes)

Main Workout:

1. **Barbell or Dumbbell Back Squat**

    o   4 sets × 8 reps

    o   Rest: 2 minutes

    o   Focus: Depth, control, bar path

2. **Romanian Deadlift**

    o   4 sets × 8 reps

    o   Rest: 2 minutes

    o   Focus: Hamstring stretch, hip hinge

3. **Bulgarian Split Squat**

    o   3 sets × 8 reps per leg

    o   Rest: 90 seconds

    o   Focus: Balance, front knee over ankle

4. **Leg Press (or Goblet Squat)**

    o   3 sets × 12 reps

    o   Rest: 90 seconds

    o   Focus: Full range of motion

5. **Single-Leg RDL**

    o   3 sets × 8 reps per leg

    o   Rest: 60 seconds

- Focus: Balance, hip hinge, hamstring engagement

6. **Plank with Shoulder Taps**

   - 3 sets × 10 taps per side
   - Rest: 60 seconds

Cool-Down (5 minutes)

[Strength Training - Day 2: Upper Push Focus]

Warm-Up (10 minutes)

Main Workout:

1. **Barbell or Dumbbell Bench Press**

   - 4 sets × 8 reps
   - Rest: 2 minutes
   - Focus: Controlled descent, drive through chest

2. **Overhead Press (Barbell or Dumbbell)**

   - 4 sets × 8 reps
   - Rest: 2 minutes
   - Focus: Vertical bar path, stable core

3. **Incline Dumbbell Press**

   - 3 sets × 10 reps
   - Rest: 90 seconds
   - Focus: Upper chest engagement

4. **Dips (Assisted if Needed)**

   - 3 sets × 8-10 reps
   - Rest: 90 seconds
   - Focus: Full range, shoulder health

5. **Lateral Raises**

   - 3 sets × 12 reps
   - Rest: 60 seconds
   - Focus: Control, no momentum

168

6. **Push-Up Holds (Top or Bottom Position)**

   o   3 sets × 20-30 seconds

   o   Rest: 60 seconds

Cool-Down (5 minutes)

[Strength Training - Day 3: Upper Pull Focus]

Warm-Up (10 minutes)

Main Workout:

1. **Pull-Ups or Lat Pulldown**

   o   4 sets × 6-10 reps

   o   Rest: 2 minutes

   o   Focus: Full range, shoulder blade retraction

2. **Barbell or Dumbbell Row**

   o   4 sets × 8 reps

   o   Rest: 2 minutes

   o   Focus: Pull to sternum, elbows back

3. **Single-Arm Dumbbell Row**

   o   3 sets × 10 reps per arm

   o   Rest: 90 seconds

   o   Focus: Minimize rotation, pull with elbow

4. **Face Pulls**

   o   3 sets × 15 reps

   o   Rest: 60 seconds

   o   Focus: Rear delts, external rotation

5. **Bicep Curls**

   o   3 sets × 10 reps

   o   Rest: 60 seconds

   o   Focus: Control, full range

6. **Hanging Knee Raises (or Dead Hang)**

169

- 3 sets × 8-12 reps (or 20-30 seconds)
- Rest: 60 seconds

Cool-Down (5 minutes)

[Optional Strength Training - Day 4: Full Body Accessory]

This fourth session is optional. Include it if you're recovering well and have time. Skip it if life is busy or you're fatigued.

Main Workout (45 minutes):

1. **Goblet Squat**: 3 sets × 12 reps
2. **Dumbbell RDL**: 3 sets × 10 reps
3. **Push-Ups**: 3 sets × 12 reps
4. **Dumbbell Row**: 3 sets × 10 reps per arm
5. **Farmer's Carry**: 3 sets × 40 seconds
6. **Pallof Press**: 3 sets × 10 per side

[Zone 2 Cardio - Week 5]

- Session 1: 45 minutes
- Session 2: 45 minutes
- Session 3: 55 minutes

[Mobility - Week 5] Continue daily routine from Phase 1.

Week 6: High-Intensity Introduction

Strength Training: Same as Week 5. Increase weight by 5-10% if you completed all reps with good form.

Zone 2 Cardio:

- Session 1: 50 minutes
- Session 2: 50 minutes

High-Intensity Interval Training (HIIT) - Week 6: Replace one Zone 2 session with HIIT.

[HIIT Session: Bike or Rower Intervals]

Warm-Up: 10 minutes easy pace

Intervals:

- 4 rounds of: 3 minutes hard effort (80-85% max heart rate), 3 minutes easy recovery

Cool-Down: 5 minutes easy pace

Total Time: 35 minutes

Notes: Hard effort means you cannot hold a conversation but can sustain the pace for the full 3 minutes. This is not all-out sprinting.

Mobility: Continue daily routine.

Week 7: Capacity Peak

Strength Training: Same exercises as Week 5. Maintain or slightly increase weight. Focus on quality reps and maintaining form under fatigue.

Zone 2 Cardio:

- Session 1: 55 minutes
- Session 2: 55 minutes

HIIT Session:

- 5 rounds of: 3 minutes hard effort, 3 minutes recovery
- Total: 40 minutes including warm-up and cool-down

Mobility: Continue daily routine. Add foam rolling for 5-10 minutes 2-3 times this week.

Week 8: Deload

Strength Training: Same exercises. Reduce to 3 sets. Reduce weight by 30%. Focus on movement quality and feeling refreshed.

Zone 2 Cardio:

- Session 1: 35 minutes (easy)
- Session 2: 35 minutes (easy)

No HIIT this week.

Mobility: Continue daily routine. Prioritize relaxation and recovery.

Goals:

- Optimize performance

- Test progress on key lifts

- Refine technique under heavier loads

- Prepare for long-term training continuation

Training Structure:

- Strength: 3-4 sessions per week

- Zone 2: 3 sessions per week, 45-60 minutes

- HIIT: 1 session per week

- Mobility: Daily

Week 9: Intensity Focus

[Strength Training - Day 1: Lower Power]

Main Workout:

1. **Barbell Back Squat**

   o 5 sets × 5 reps (heavier than Phase 2)

   o Rest: 2.5-3 minutes

2. **Conventional Deadlift (or Trap Bar Deadlift)**

   o 4 sets × 5 reps

   o Rest: 2.5-3 minutes

3. **Front Squat (or Goblet Squat)**

   o 3 sets × 8 reps

   o Rest: 2 minutes

4. **Walking Lunges**

   o 3 sets × 10 reps per leg

   o Rest: 90 seconds

5. **Glute-Ham Raise (or Nordic Curl)**

- o   3 sets × 6-8 reps

- o   Rest: 90 seconds

6. **Pallof Press**

- o   3 sets × 10 per side

[Strength Training - Day 2: Upper Power]

Main Workout:

1. **Barbell Bench Press**

    - o   5 sets × 5 reps

    - o   Rest: 2.5-3 minutes

2. **Weighted Pull-Ups (or Lat Pulldown)**

    - o   4 sets × 6-8 reps

    - o   Rest: 2.5 minutes

3. **Overhead Press**

    - o   4 sets × 6 reps

    - o   Rest: 2 minutes

4. **Incline Dumbbell Press**

    - o   3 sets × 8 reps

    - o   Rest: 90 seconds

5. **Cable or Band Row**

    - o   3 sets × 12 reps

    - o   Rest: 90 seconds

6. **Hanging Leg Raises**

    - o   3 sets × 10 reps

[Strength Training - Day 3: Full Body Strength]

Main Workout:

1. **Trap Bar Deadlift (or RDL)**

    - o   5 sets × 5 reps

o   Rest: 2.5 minutes

2. **Bulgarian Split Squat**

      o   4 sets × 6 reps per leg

      o   Rest: 2 minutes

3. **Weighted Dips**

      o   4 sets × 8 reps

      o   Rest: 2 minutes

4. **Single-Arm Dumbbell Row**

      o   4 sets × 8 reps per arm

      o   Rest: 90 seconds

5. **Farmer's Carry (Heavy)**

      o   4 sets × 30-40 seconds

      o   Rest: 2 minutes

6. **Plank Hold (Weighted if Possible)**

      o   3 sets × 30-45 seconds

Zone 2 Cardio:

- Session 1: 50 minutes

- Session 2: 50 minutes

HIIT:

- 6 rounds: 2 minutes hard, 2 minutes recovery

Mobility: Daily routine.

Week 10: Volume Peak

Strength Training: Same exercises as Week 9. Increase sets to 5-6 for main lifts (exercises 1-2). This is the highest volume week of the program.

Zone 2:

- Session 1: 55 minutes

- Session 2: 55 minutes

HIIT:

- 6 rounds: 2.5 minutes hard, 2.5 minutes recovery

Mobility: Daily routine plus 2-3 foam rolling sessions.

Week 11: Testing Preparation

Strength Training: Same exercises. Reduce sets to 3-4. Reduce volume by 30% to prepare for testing week. Focus on crispness and speed of movement.

Zone 2:

- Session 1: 45 minutes

- Session 2: 45 minutes

HIIT:

- 4 rounds: 3 minutes hard, 3 minutes recovery (moderate week)

Mobility: Daily routine.

Week 12: Testing & Celebration

[Strength Testing Week]

Day 1: Lower Body Test

- Warm up thoroughly

- Work up to heavy 3-5 rep max on squat and deadlift

- Test your progress from Week 1

Day 2: Upper Body Test

- Warm up thoroughly

- Work up to heavy 3-5 rep max on bench press and weighted pull-up

- Test your progress from Week 1

Day 3: Optional Accessory Work

- Light, fun session

- Focus on movements you enjoy

Zone 2:

- Session 1: 40 minutes (easy, celebratory)

- Session 2: 40 minutes (easy)

Optional HIIT:

- Perform a final test: 1-mile run for time, 2K row, or 5-minute max distance on bike

- Record results for future comparison

Mobility: Continue daily routine.

You've completed 12 weeks. You're stronger, fitter, and more capable than when you started. You've built habits, movement patterns, and capacity that will serve you for years.

What's Next?

You have three options:

1. **Repeat the program** with heavier weights and better technique

2. **Create a maintenance phase** using Week 9's structure indefinitely

3. **Design your own program** using the principles you've learned

The program ends, but the practice continues. Training for longevity is not a 12-week project. It's a lifelong commitment. You now have the tools, the knowledge, and the experience to train for decades.

Record your progress. Celebrate your wins. Then keep moving forward.

CHAPTER 14: CARDIO FOR LONGEVITY

Cardiovascular training is misunderstood. Most people equate cardio with suffering: breathless intervals, monotonous treadmill sessions, or endless running. They do it to burn calories or lose weight, then wonder why they hate it and quit.

Longevity-focused cardio is different. It's about building mitochondrial function, improving metabolic health, and creating the aerobic base that allows you to sustain effort without fatigue. Done correctly, it feels sustainable, even enjoyable.

This chapter explains Zone 2 training, how to know you're doing it right without expensive equipment, and which modalities work best for long-term consistency.

Zone 2 Details

Zone 2 is the intensity at which your body primarily uses fat for fuel while producing energy aerobically. It's the sweet spot where you build mitochondrial capacity, improve insulin sensitivity, and enhance fat oxidation without accumulating fatigue.

Physiological Markers:

- Heart rate: Approximately 60-70% of maximum

- Lactate: Below 2 mmol/L (you won't measure this, but it's the scientific marker)

- Breathing: Nasal breathing comfortable, conversation possible but not easy

- Perceived effort: 3-4 out of 10

At this intensity, your mitochondria work efficiently. You're producing ATP aerobically, meaning with oxygen and without significant lactate buildup. You can sustain this pace for hours if needed.

Why Zone 2 Matters: Most people skip Zone 2 entirely. They either train too easy (Zone 1, barely elevated heart rate) or too hard (Zone 3-4, breathless and accumulating fatigue). Zone 2 requires discipline because it feels almost too easy, yet it's where the magic happens.

Zone 2 training improves:

- Mitochondrial density and efficiency

- Fat oxidation capacity

- Insulin sensitivity

- Lactate clearance

- Aerobic base for all other training

Think of Zone 2 as building the engine. Without it, your cardiovascular system has no foundation for higher-intensity work or sustained daily activity.

Training Volume: Target 150-180 minutes per week, split into 3-4 sessions. A typical week might include:

- Session 1: 45 minutes

- Session 2: 50 minutes

- Session 3: 60 minutes

- Total: 155 minutes

More is not always better. Excessive Zone 2 can interfere with strength training recovery. The goal is enough to drive adaptation without exceeding recovery capacity.

How to Know You're in Zone 2 Without Gadgets

You don't need a heart rate monitor or lactate meter to train effectively in Zone 2. Your body provides clear feedback.

The Talk Test: This is the simplest and most reliable method. At Zone 2 intensity, you should be able to speak in full sentences, but with slight difficulty. You could hold a conversation, but you wouldn't want to give a speech. You definitely cannot sing.

If you can talk easily and comfortably, you're likely in Zone 1 (too easy). If you can only speak a few words at a time, you're in Zone 3 or higher (too hard).

The Nasal Breathing Test: Try breathing only through your nose. If you can maintain nasal breathing comfortably for several minutes, you're likely in Zone 2. If you're gasping for air or must switch to mouth breathing immediately, you're working too hard.

Nasal breathing naturally regulates intensity. Your nose cannot deliver as much oxygen as your mouth, which forces you to slow down to a sustainable pace.

Perceived Exertion: On a scale of 1-10, Zone 2 should feel like a 3-4. It's noticeably harder than walking around your house, but you're not suffering. You could maintain this pace for an hour or more without dreading every minute.

If it feels hard, like you're pushing, you're too high. If it feels like you're barely working, you're too low.

Heart Rate Formula (If You Have a Monitor): Calculate your estimated maximum heart rate: 220 minus your age. Zone 2 is approximately 60-70% of that number.

Example for a 45-year-old:

- Max HR: 220 - 45 = 175

- Zone 2: 105-122 bpm

This formula is imprecise but gives a reasonable target range. Use the talk test and breathing to fine-tune.

Common Mistakes: Most people train too hard. They feel like they should be working harder, so they push into Zone 3. This defeats the purpose. Zone 2 requires humility. Let go of ego and train at the right intensity, even if it feels easy.

Walking, Cycling, Rowing, Swimming Options

The best cardio modality is the one you'll do consistently. Choose based on preference, accessibility, and joint health.

Walking: The most accessible and joint-friendly option. Walking is underrated. A brisk walk at a pace where you're breathing harder than normal but can still talk is often perfect Zone 2.

Benefits:

- Zero equipment needed

- Can be done anywhere

- Very low injury risk

- Easy to integrate into daily life

Guidelines:

- Walk at a pace of 3.5-4.5 mph on flat ground, or slower uphill

- Swing arms naturally

- Focus on posture: head up, shoulders back

- Increase intensity with hills or incline rather than speed

Cycling: Excellent for people with knee or hip issues. Cycling removes impact while allowing high training volumes.

Benefits:

- Low joint stress

- Can cover long distances

- Easy to maintain consistent intensity

- Outdoor or indoor options

Guidelines:

- Maintain steady cadence (70-90 rpm)

- Keep resistance moderate, not so hard you're grinding

- Outdoor cycling: choose relatively flat routes for Zone 2

- Indoor cycling: use fan for cooling, avoid high-intensity spin classes

Rowing: Full-body cardio that builds strength and endurance simultaneously. Rowing engages legs, core, and upper body.

Benefits:

- Full-body engagement

- Low impact

- Builds posterior chain strength

- Efficient time use

Guidelines:

- Focus on technique: legs drive, hips extend, then arms pull

- Maintain steady pace (18-22 strokes per minute for Zone 2)

- Don't go too hard; rowing tempts people to push intensity

- Keep damper setting at 3-5 for aerobic work

Swimming: Ideal for people with joint issues or injuries. Swimming is non-impact and cooling, making it sustainable for long durations.

Benefits:

- Zero impact

- Cooling (prevents overheating)

- Technical skill development

- Full-body conditioning

Guidelines:

- Choose strokes you can sustain: freestyle or backstroke typically work best

- Focus on smooth, rhythmic breathing

- Rest 10-15 seconds at the end of each lap if needed to stay in Zone 2

- Consider water jogging or aqua aerobics as alternatives

Elliptical/Stair Climber: Good gym-based options when weather or time constraints limit outdoor activity.

Benefits:

- Controlled environment

- Adjustable resistance

- Low impact (elliptical)

- Consistent intensity

Guidelines:

- Avoid the trap of watching TV and zoning out—maintain proper intensity

- Elliptical: keep resistance moderate, don't just flail your legs

- Stair climber: maintain upright posture, don't lean heavily on rails

Choosing Your Modality: Variety is beneficial. Rotating between modalities prevents overuse injuries and maintains interest. A typical week might include:

- Monday: 45-minute walk

- Wednesday: 50-minute bike ride

- Saturday: 60-minute row

Or stick with one modality if you prefer consistency. Both approaches work.

Zone 2 cardio is the foundation of cardiovascular longevity. It's not glamorous, it's not intense, and it won't leave you drenched in sweat. But it works. It builds mitochondrial function, improves metabolic health, and creates the aerobic base that supports everything else you do.

The talk test and nasal breathing are your guides. Use them to stay honest about intensity. Most people need to slow down, not speed up.

Choose a modality you enjoy and can access consistently. Walking is always available. Cycling protects joints. Rowing builds strength. Swimming is therapeutic. Variety or consistency—both work.

Commit to 150-180 minutes per week. Break it into manageable sessions. Show up consistently. The benefits compound over months and years.

Zone 2 is patience. It's discipline. It's trusting the process when your ego wants to push harder. Master it, and you build a cardiovascular system that lasts decades.

CHAPTER 15: MOBILITY, BALANCE, & FALL PREVENTION

Strength and cardio get attention. Mobility and balance are ignored until something goes wrong. A fall. A pulled muscle. Chronic pain that won't resolve. Then suddenly, these overlooked qualities become everything.

Mobility, balance, and stability are not optional accessories to fitness. They are foundational to moving well, training consistently, and maintaining independence as you age. This chapter provides the framework for preserving and improving these qualities throughout your life.

Joint Health

Your joints are non-renewable. Once cartilage degrades, it doesn't regenerate. Once ligaments are damaged, they heal slowly and incompletely. Joint health determines whether you can train for decades or whether pain forces you to stop.

Movement as Medicine: Joints need movement to stay healthy. Cartilage has no blood supply; it receives nutrients through compression and decompression during movement. Inactivity starves cartilage. Movement feeds it.

But not all movement is beneficial. Repetitive stress, poor technique, and excessive load damage joints. The key is moving regularly through full ranges of motion with appropriate loads.

Daily Joint Maintenance: Spend 5-10 minutes daily taking your joints through their full ranges of motion:

Ankles: Circles (10 each direction per foot), dorsiflexion and plantarflexion **Knees:** Gentle bends and extensions, avoiding hyperextension **Hips:** Circles, hip openers (90/90 position), leg swings **Spine:** Cat-cow, spinal rotations, side bends **Shoulders:** Arm circles, wall slides, shoulder dislocations with band or towel

This isn't a workout. It's maintenance. Do it every morning or evening as a ritual.

Loaded Carries for Joint Stability: Farmer's carries, suitcase carries, and overhead carries build joint stability throughout the body. The weight creates compression that forces stabilizer muscles to work. This strengthens the supporting structures around joints.

Include carries in your training weekly:

- Farmer's carry: 3 sets × 40 seconds

- Suitcase carry: 3 sets × 30 seconds per side

- Overhead carry: 2 sets × 20 seconds per arm

Avoid These Joint Destroyers:

- Training through sharp pain

- Ignoring technique for heavier weight

- Excessive volume without recovery

- Repetitive movements without variation

Pain is information. Listen to it. Modify or eliminate exercises that consistently hurt. There are always alternatives.

Balance Drills

Balance declines predictably with age unless you train it. Poor balance is the primary reason older adults fall. Falls lead to fractures, hospitalizations, loss of independence, and cascading decline.

Balance is trainable at any age. The earlier you start, the better, but it's never too late.

Why Balance Declines:

- Reduced proprioception (body awareness in space)
- Weakened stabilizer muscles
- Decreased reaction time
- Vision changes
- Vestibular system decline

You can counteract all of these with specific training.

Daily Balance Practice:

Single-Leg Stance:

- Stand on one leg for 30-60 seconds
- Perform with eyes open, then progress to eyes closed
- Do this while brushing teeth or waiting for coffee

Tandem Walk:

- Walk heel-to-toe in a straight line
- 20 steps forward, 20 steps backward
- Progress to doing this on an unstable surface like a balance pad

Single-Leg Deadlift (Unweighted):

- Stand on one leg, hinge at hip, reach toward floor with opposite hand
- Return to standing
- 8 reps per leg, focusing on control and stability

Clock Reaches:

- Stand on one leg

- Reach with opposite leg to 12 o'clock, 3 o'clock, 6 o'clock positions

- Focus on maintaining stable hip and ankle

- 5 reaches to each position per leg

Integrated Balance Training: Include single-leg exercises in strength training:

- Single-leg RDL

- Bulgarian split squat

- Single-leg step-up

- Single-leg glute bridge

These build strength while simultaneously training balance and stability.

Progression: Start with stable surfaces and open eyes. Progress to:

- Eyes closed

- Unstable surfaces (foam pad, balance disc)

- Adding external load

- Adding cognitive tasks (count backward while balancing)

Balance training should feel challenging but safe. Stay near a wall or sturdy surface when learning.

Aging-Proofing Movement

Certain movement patterns become difficult or impossible if you don't maintain them. The ability to get up from the floor, squat deeply, reach overhead, and rotate your spine are all use-it-or-lose-it capacities.

The Sit-Rise Test: This simple test predicts longevity. Can you sit down on the floor and stand back up without using your hands, knees, or forearms for support?

Scoring:

- Start with 10 points

- Lose 1 point for each support used (hand, knee, forearm, side of leg)

- Lose 0.5 points for visible instability

Studies show people who score 8 or higher have significantly lower mortality risk than those who score 3 or lower. This test measures strength, flexibility, balance, and coordination simultaneously.

Practice this movement monthly. If you can't do it now, work toward it by:

- Practicing getting up from progressively lower surfaces

- Building hip and ankle mobility

- Strengthening legs and core

Deep Squat Hold: The ability to squat with feet flat on the ground, knees and hips fully flexed, is a fundamental human position. Many adults lose this capacity through disuse.

Practice:

- Hold a deep squat for 30-60 seconds daily

- Use a support (doorframe, pole) if needed initially

- Focus on keeping heels down and torso upright

- Over time, reduce support and increase duration

Floor Work: Spend time on the floor daily:

- Sit in various positions: cross-legged, 90/90, kneeling

- Practice transitioning between positions

- Get up and down from the floor multiple times

This builds hip mobility, core strength, and comfort with floor-based movement.

Overhead Reach: Can you reach fully overhead with straight arms, without arching your lower back excessively? This requires shoulder mobility and thoracic extension.

Practice:

- Wall slides: Stand with back against wall, slide arms overhead

- Overhead stretches with doorframe

- Light overhead pressing in your strength training

Spinal Rotation: The ability to rotate your spine is essential for daily activities: looking over your shoulder while driving, reaching behind you, getting dressed.

Practice:

- Seated spinal rotations: 10 reps each direction

- Thoracic rotation in quadruped position

- Include rotational exercises in training (woodchops, medicine ball throws)

Get Up, Get Down: Practice the Turkish get-up movement (doesn't need to be weighted). This complex movement builds strength, mobility, and coordination through multiple planes of motion.

Simplified version:

- Lie on your back

- Roll to your side

- Push up to seated

- Come to kneeling

- Stand up

- Reverse the sequence to return to lying down

Do this 2-3 times per week, alternating sides.

Mobility, balance, and movement quality determine whether you can train consistently now and maintain independence later. These qualities don't develop from strength and cardio alone. They require specific, deliberate practice.

Joint health requires daily maintenance, not heroic efforts. Five minutes of movement each morning preserves the freedom to move without pain.

Balance must be trained, not assumed. Single-leg work, balance drills, and proprioceptive challenges prevent the falls that end independence for millions of older adults.

Movement capacity must be maintained through use. If you don't regularly squat, get up from the floor, reach overhead, and rotate your spine, you will lose these abilities. By the time you need them desperately, it's too late.

Integrate these practices into daily life:

- Morning joint mobility routine

- Balance practice while brushing teeth

- Floor time in the evening

- Movement quality checks during training

This is not extra work. It's insurance. It's the difference between moving freely at eighty and being afraid to leave your chair.

Your future self will thank you for the time you invest now.

CHAPTER 16: SLEEP AS A LONGEVITY TOOL

Sleep is not optional. It's not something you sacrifice to get more done. It's not a weakness or luxury. Sleep is the foundation upon which everything else is built.

Without adequate sleep, your training doesn't produce adaptation. Your nutrition doesn't support recovery. Your stress tolerance collapses. Your metabolic health deteriorates. Your longevity shortens.

This chapter explains what sleep does, why consistency matters more than perfection, and how to build routines that support deep, restorative rest.

Sleep Architecture Basics

Sleep is not a uniform state. Your brain cycles through distinct stages, each serving specific functions.

NREM Sleep (Non-Rapid Eye Movement):

Stage 1: Light sleep, transition from wakefulness (5% of night) **Stage 2:** Deeper sleep, memory consolidation begins (45% of night) **Stage 3:** Deep sleep (slow-wave sleep), physical recovery, growth hormone release (25% of night)

Deep sleep is when your body repairs tissue, strengthens immune function, and clears metabolic waste from the brain. This is the most restorative stage.

REM Sleep (Rapid Eye Movement): REM sleep is when you dream. It's critical for emotional regulation, memory consolidation, and cognitive function (25% of night).

Sleep Cycles: You cycle through these stages approximately every 90 minutes. A full night contains 4-6 cycles. Waking during a cycle feels groggier than waking between cycles.

What Sleep Does:

- **Physical recovery:** Muscle repair, tissue growth, immune strengthening

- **Metabolic regulation:** Insulin sensitivity, appetite hormone balance, glucose regulation

- **Cognitive function:** Memory consolidation, learning, problem-solving

- **Emotional regulation:** Stress processing, mood stabilization

- **Waste clearance:** Glymphatic system clears metabolic waste from brain

Chronic sleep deprivation impairs all of these functions. Even one night of poor sleep reduces insulin sensitivity, increases hunger hormones, impairs cognitive performance, and reduces training adaptation.

How Much Sleep: Most adults need 7-9 hours. Individual needs vary, but virtually no one thrives on six hours or less. If you need an alarm to wake up, you're not getting enough sleep.

Consistency Over Perfection

Sleep quality varies. Some nights you'll sleep deeply. Other nights you'll wake repeatedly. Life disrupts sleep: travel, stress, illness, a crying baby.

Perfection is impossible. Consistency is achievable.

Consistent Sleep Schedule: Go to bed and wake up at the same time every day, including weekends. Your body has a circadian rhythm that thrives on predictability.

When you vary sleep times dramatically (staying up late Friday and Saturday, sleeping in Sunday), you create social jet lag. Your circadian rhythm gets confused, sleep quality suffers, and you feel worse all week.

Target a consistent schedule within 30-60 minutes. If you typically sleep 10:30 PM to 6:30 AM, don't suddenly stay up until 1 AM or sleep until 10 AM.

Sleep Debt is Real: You cannot "catch up" on sleep by sleeping 10 hours once. Chronic sleep deprivation accumulates. One good night doesn't erase weeks of five-hour nights.

Prioritize consistency. Seven hours every night is far better than five hours six days and ten hours one day.

Don't Obsess: Sleep tracking devices are useful but can create anxiety. If you're checking your sleep score every morning and stressing about it, the device is making things worse.

Focus on how you feel:

- Do you wake naturally without an alarm?

- Do you feel rested during the day?

- Can you focus without excessive caffeine?

- Do you fall asleep within 15-20 minutes?

If yes, your sleep is probably adequate, regardless of what your tracker says.

Pre-Sleep Routines

What you do in the hour before bed determines how quickly you fall asleep and how well you sleep.

Wind-Down Ritual (60-90 Minutes Before Bed):

Dim the lights: Bright light signals daytime to your brain. Reduce lighting intensity throughout your home. Use lamps instead of overhead lights.

Avoid screens: Blue light from phones, tablets, and computers suppresses melatonin production. If you must use screens, use blue-light blocking glasses or apps that reduce blue light.

Cool down: Your body temperature needs to drop to fall asleep. Take a warm shower or bath 60-90 minutes before bed. The subsequent cooling helps trigger sleep.

Light reading or stretching: Engage in calm, non-stimulating activities. Reading physical books, gentle stretching, or light mobility work all signal your body to wind down.

Avoid stimulating content: Don't watch intense movies, read disturbing news, or engage in heated discussions. Your nervous system needs to calm, not activate.

Pre-Sleep Routine Template:

9:00 PM: Dim lights throughout home 9:15 PM: Warm shower 9:30 PM: Light stretching or foam rolling (5-10 minutes) 9:45 PM: Read in bed with low lighting 10:15 PM: Lights out

This routine signals your body that sleep is approaching. Consistency trains your brain to prepare for sleep automatically.

What to Avoid:

Large meals: Finish eating 2-3 hours before bed. Digestion interferes with sleep quality.

Intense exercise: Training raises cortisol and body temperature, making sleep difficult. Finish workouts at least 3 hours before bed. Light movement (walking, stretching) is fine.

Alcohol: While alcohol makes you drowsy initially, it fragments sleep and reduces REM. Avoid alcohol within 3 hours of bed.

Arguments or stressful conversations: Save difficult discussions for earlier in the day.

Light, Caffeine, Alcohol Considerations

Light Exposure:

Morning light: Get bright light exposure within 30 minutes of waking. Go outside for 10-15 minutes or sit by a window. Morning light sets your circadian rhythm and improves nighttime sleep.

Daytime light: Spend time outdoors during the day. Natural light exposure keeps your circadian rhythm strong.

Evening darkness: Reduce light exposure as evening progresses. Dim lights starting 2 hours before bed. Blackout curtains or eye masks help if your room isn't dark enough.

Caffeine:

Caffeine has a half-life of 5-6 hours. If you consume 200mg of caffeine at 2 PM, 100mg is still in your system at 8 PM. Even if you fall asleep, caffeine reduces deep sleep quality.

Guidelines:

- Stop caffeine intake 8-10 hours before bed

- If you sleep at 10 PM, last caffeine by noon or 2 PM

- Be aware of hidden sources: chocolate, some medications, green tea

Individual sensitivity varies. Some people metabolize caffeine quickly. Others are highly sensitive. Experiment to find your cutoff time.

Alcohol:

Alcohol is one of the worst substances for sleep quality. It acts as a sedative, helping you fall asleep quickly, but it prevents deep sleep and REM sleep. You wake frequently, often unaware, resulting in fragmented, unrestorative sleep.

If you drink:

- Finish alcohol 3-4 hours before bed minimum

- Limit quantity: 1-2 drinks maximum

- Hydrate: drink water between alcoholic drinks

The best choice for sleep is no alcohol in the evening. If sleep quality is poor and you drink regularly at night, eliminating alcohol is the single most impactful change you can make.

Sleep is non-negotiable. It's the foundation of recovery, metabolic health, cognitive function, and longevity. Without it, everything else suffers.

You cannot train your way out of poor sleep. You cannot eat your way out of it. You cannot supplement your way around it. There is no substitute.

Prioritize consistency: same sleep and wake times daily. Build a wind-down routine that signals your body to prepare for rest. Manage light exposure: bright in the morning, dim in the evening. Cut caffeine early. Minimize or eliminate evening alcohol.

Sleep is not time wasted. It's the time when your body rebuilds, your brain consolidates learning, and your system resets. It's when adaptation from training actually occurs.

If you only make one change from this book, improve your sleep. Everything else becomes easier when you're well-rested.

CHAPTER 17: STRESS, HORMONES & RECOVERY

Stress is not the enemy. Stress is the stimulus for adaptation. Training is stress. Learning is stress. Challenge is stress. Without stress, there is no growth.

But chronic, unmanaged stress is destructive. It disrupts hormones, impairs recovery, accelerates aging, and undermines every effort you make to improve health.

This chapter explains how stress affects your body, how to balance your nervous system, and practical tools for managing stress and building emotional resilience.

Nervous System Balance

Your autonomic nervous system has two branches:

Sympathetic (Fight or Flight): Activated during stress, exercise, or threat. Increases heart rate, blood pressure, cortisol, and alertness. Prepares body for action.

Parasympathetic (Rest and Digest): Activated during rest, recovery, and safety. Decreases heart rate, promotes digestion, supports tissue repair and recovery.

Both are essential. The problem arises when you're stuck in sympathetic dominance: constantly stressed, never fully relaxed, always "on." This is the modern condition.

Signs of Chronic Sympathetic Dominance:

- Difficulty falling asleep or staying asleep

- Elevated resting heart rate

- Persistent fatigue despite rest

- Digestive issues

- Frequent illness

- Irritability and mood swings

- Reduced training performance

Restoring Balance: You must actively engage the parasympathetic system. It doesn't happen automatically just because you stop working.

Practices that activate parasympathetic response:

- Deep breathing exercises

- Meditation or quiet sitting

- Time in nature

- Gentle movement (walking, yoga)

- Social connection with trusted people

- Massage or bodywork

- Laughter and play

These aren't luxuries. They're physiological necessities for recovery and health.

Breathwork Basics

Breathing is the most accessible tool for nervous system regulation. You can shift from stressed to calm in minutes using specific breathing patterns.

Why Breathing Works: Your breath is directly connected to your autonomic nervous system. Slow, deep breathing with extended exhales activates the vagus nerve, which triggers parasympathetic response.

Box Breathing (Stress Reduction):

- Inhale for 4 seconds

- Hold for 4 seconds

- Exhale for 4 seconds

- Hold for 4 seconds

- Repeat for 5 minutes

Use this before bed, after stressful events, or anytime you feel activated and need to calm down.

4-7-8 Breathing (Sleep Preparation):

- Inhale through nose for 4 seconds

- Hold for 7 seconds

- Exhale through mouth for 8 seconds

- Repeat 4-8 times

The extended exhale strongly activates parasympathetic response. This is excellent before sleep.

Physiological Sigh (Immediate Stress Relief):

- Double inhale through nose (inhale, then quick second inhale to fill lungs completely)

- Long, slow exhale through mouth

One or two cycles immediately reduces stress and lowers heart rate. Use in real-time during stressful moments.

Daily Practice: Spend 5-10 minutes daily on breathwork. Morning or evening, build it into your routine like brushing teeth. Consistency creates a baseline of nervous system resilience.

Mental Recovery

Physical recovery gets attention. Mental recovery is ignored, yet it's equally important. Your brain needs downtime to process information, consolidate learning, and restore cognitive capacity.

Cognitive Load: Every decision, every task, every interaction requires mental energy. Cognitive load accumulates throughout the day. When it exceeds your capacity, performance collapses.

Active Mental Recovery Practices:

Meditation (5-20 minutes daily): Sit quietly. Focus on breath. When mind wanders, gently return to breath. This isn't about stopping thoughts. It's about training attention and creating space from constant mental activity.

Nature Exposure: Time in nature reduces cortisol, lowers blood pressure, and restores attention. Even 20 minutes in a park improves mood and cognitive function. Aim for daily nature exposure when possible.

Digital Detox: Constant connectivity fragments attention. Set boundaries: no phone for first hour after waking, no screens after 8 PM, one full day per week with minimal screen time.

Monotasking: Stop trying to do multiple things simultaneously. Focus on one task at a time. Complete it. Move to the next. This reduces cognitive load and improves quality.

Downtime: Allow yourself to do nothing. Sit. Stare out the window. Let your mind wander. Boredom is not a problem to solve. It's necessary for creativity and restoration.

Mental Recovery Schedule:

- Morning: 10 minutes meditation
- Midday: 15-minute walk outside
- Evening: 30 minutes reading (physical book, not screens)
- Weekly: Half-day with no digital devices

Mental recovery isn't laziness. It's maintenance of the most important tool you have.

Emotional Resilience

Emotional resilience is the ability to experience difficult emotions without being overwhelmed by them, to face setbacks without collapsing, and to maintain perspective during challenges.

It's not about being tough or suppressing feelings. It's about having the capacity to feel, process, and move through emotions without being consumed by them.

Building Emotional Resilience:

Acknowledge emotions: Don't suppress or ignore difficult feelings. Notice them, name them, allow them to exist. "I'm feeling anxious about this presentation" is more useful than "I'm fine."

Separate feeling from identity: You're not your emotions. You're experiencing an emotion. "I feel angry" is different from "I am angry." This creates space between you and the feeling.

Develop perspective: Ask: "Will this matter in a year? In five years?" Most daily stresses lose importance with temporal distance.

Build support systems: Emotional resilience isn't rugged individualism. It's having trusted people you can talk to honestly. Connection is protective. Isolation is corrosive.

Practice self-compassion: Treat yourself with the same kindness you'd offer a friend. You will make mistakes. You will fail. You will struggle. This is being human, not being defective.

Maintain routines during stress: When life is chaotic, routines provide stability. Keep training, eating well, and sleeping consistently even when everything else is uncertain.

Resilience is a Practice: You build emotional resilience the same way you build physical capacity: through repeated exposure to manageable stress with adequate recovery. Each time you face difficulty and come through it, you grow stronger.

Avoid both extremes: don't avoid all discomfort, but don't chronically overwhelm yourself. Find the edge where you're challenged but not broken.

Stress is inevitable. How you manage it determines whether it builds you up or breaks you down.

Balance your nervous system through breathwork, meditation, nature exposure, and genuine rest. Don't stay activated constantly. Actively engage recovery practices daily.

Prioritize mental recovery as seriously as physical recovery. Your brain needs downtime. Protect it from constant stimulation and decision-making.

Build emotional resilience through awareness, perspective, connection, and self-compassion. You will face challenges. Resilience determines whether they strengthen or diminish you.

Recovery is not passive. It's not just the absence of training. It's active practices that restore your nervous system, mental capacity, and emotional reserves.

Without recovery, stress accumulates until something breaks. With intentional recovery practices, stress becomes the stimulus for growth rather than the cause of breakdown.

Train hard. Recover harder. Both matter equally.

CONCLUSION

PRACTICE, NOT PERFECTION

You have reached the end of this book, but not the end of the practice.

Everything in these pages—the nutrition principles, the recipes, the training program, the recovery strategies—is simply a map. The territory is your life. The map shows you where to go, but you must walk the path yourself.

And that path is not straight. It never is.

Long-Term Mindset

Longevity is not a twelve-week project. It is not a New Year's resolution that fades by February. It is not a goal you achieve and then stop working toward.

Longevity is a practice that spans decades. It is the accumulation of thousands of small decisions, repeated consistently over time, that compound into something extraordinary.

Think in Decades, Not Days:

The choices you make today are shaping the body you will inhabit at seventy, eighty, and beyond. That training session you're tempted to skip matters. That meal you're about to eat matters. That sleep you're sacrificing matters. Not because any single choice is catastrophic, but because the pattern of choices creates your trajectory.

One missed workout means nothing. A pattern of missed workouts over months means everything.

One poor meal changes nothing. A pattern of poor eating over years changes everything.

This is both humbling and empowering. You cannot undo years of neglect with one heroic effort. But you can change your trajectory starting today, and over time, that change becomes transformation.

Embrace the Plateau:

Progress is not linear. You will experience periods of rapid improvement followed by long plateaus where nothing seems to change. This is normal. This is expected. This is when most people quit.

The plateau is not failure. It is consolidation. Your body is adapting, integrating, and preparing for the next phase of growth. Trust the process during the plateau. Keep showing up. Keep doing the work. The breakthrough comes when you least expect it.

Longevity training is not about constant progress. It is about consistent practice. Some years you will get stronger. Other years you will simply maintain. Both are victories.

Redefine Success:

Success is not a number on the scale, a weight on the bar, or a time on the clock. Success is showing up consistently. Success is training at sixty the same way you trained at forty. Success is moving without pain. Success is independence at eighty.

Measure success by what you can do, not by how you compare to others. Measure it by consistency, not perfection. Measure it by the quality of your life, not the aesthetics of your body.

Zoom Out:

When you feel discouraged, zoom out. One bad week means nothing in the context of a year. One bad month means nothing in the context of a decade. What matters is the overall trend, the general direction, the pattern over time.

Are you stronger this year than you were five years ago? Are you more capable? More resilient? More consistent? If yes, you are winning. If no, adjust. But don't let short-term setbacks obscure long-term progress.

The long-term mindset protects you from the despair of temporary failure and the arrogance of temporary success. Both are fleeting. The practice is what endures.

Identity-Based Habits

Behavior change fails when it focuses on outcomes. "I want to lose twenty pounds." "I want to run a marathon." "I want to look better." These are outcome goals, and they're fragile. Once achieved, motivation disappears. Once the goal is missed, you quit.

Identity-based habits work differently. They focus not on what you want to achieve, but on who you want to become.

Shift from Outcome to Identity:

Instead of: "I want to lose weight." Think: "I am someone who takes care of my body."

Instead of: "I need to work out more." Think: "I am someone who trains."

Instead of: "I should eat healthier." Think: "I am someone who nourishes my body with quality food."

The language shift is subtle but powerful. When behavior aligns with identity, it becomes automatic. You don't have to force yourself to train. You train because that's who you are. You don't have to resist junk food. You don't eat it because it doesn't align with who you are.

Build Identity Through Action:

Identity is not something you declare. It is something you prove to yourself through action. Every time you train, you cast a vote for the identity "I am someone who trains." Every time you choose a protein-rich meal, you cast a vote for "I am someone who eats well."

The more votes you cast, the stronger the identity becomes. Eventually, the identity becomes self-reinforcing. You don't think about whether to train. You just train. It's what you do.

Start small. Cast one vote today. Then another tomorrow. Then another. Over time, these votes accumulate into an identity that carries you forward even when motivation fades.

Protect Your Identity During Setbacks:

You will miss workouts. You will eat poorly. You will fall off the path. This is inevitable. The question is not whether you will slip, but how you respond when you do.

Don't let a missed workout become a missed week. Don't let one poor meal become a poor month. Return to your identity as quickly as possible.

"I am someone who trains" doesn't mean you never miss a workout. It means that when you do, you return to training at the next opportunity without spiraling into self-criticism or abandonment.

Identity-based habits are resilient because they don't rely on perfection. They rely on consistency over time. Imperfect action, repeated, builds the identity stronger than perfect action done once.

You Become What You Practice:

If you practice training, you become a person who trains. If you practice eating well, you become a person who eats well. If you practice recovery, you become a person who recovers well.

The practice shapes the identity. The identity reinforces the practice. This is the virtuous cycle that makes longevity sustainable.

Who do you want to be at seventy? At eighty? Start being that person today. Cast votes for that identity with every choice you make. Over time, the gap between who you are and who you want to be disappears.

Aging with Capability

Aging is inevitable. Decline is not.

Most of what we attribute to aging is actually the result of inactivity, poor nutrition, and accumulated neglect. The frailty we see in older adults is not the natural consequence of time. It is the consequence of decades without resistance training, decades of poor metabolic health, decades of prioritizing everything except physical capacity.

You do not have to age that way.

Capability as the Goal:

The goal of longevity training is not to look young. It is to remain capable. Capability means:

- Standing up from the floor without assistance
- Carrying your groceries without strain
- Climbing stairs without breathlessness
- Playing with grandchildren without pain
- Traveling without exhaustion
- Living independently without fear

These are not trivial goals. These are the markers of a life well-lived. These are the reasons to train.

Aging Is Not an Excuse:

"I'm too old to start strength training." "I'm too old to change my diet." "I'm too old to improve."

These statements are false. Age is not a barrier to improvement. It is simply a variable that influences the rate of progress.

Can you gain as much muscle at seventy as you could at thirty? No. But you can gain muscle at seventy. You can get stronger. You can improve cardiovascular fitness. You can enhance mobility and balance. The body remains responsive to training stimulus throughout life.

The research is clear: resistance training builds muscle in octogenarians. Cardiovascular training improves VO_2 max in septuagenarians. Mobility work enhances range of motion at any age.

It is never too late to start. It is never too late to improve. The only time it's too late is when you stop trying.

Adjust Expectations, Not Effort:

As you age, recovery takes longer. Injuries heal more slowly. Adaptation requires more patience. This is reality. Accept it.

But acceptance does not mean resignation. It means adjusting your approach to match your current capacity while continuing to challenge yourself appropriately.

Train smarter, not necessarily harder. Prioritize technique over load. Include more recovery time. Listen to your body more carefully. But keep training. Keep moving. Keep challenging yourself.

The alternative is decline. The alternative is dependence. The alternative is watching your world shrink year by year until you can no longer do the things that matter to you.

That is not inevitable. That is a choice. Choose differently.

Model What's Possible:

Every time you train at sixty, you show others what's possible at sixty. Every time you move well at seventy, you redefine what seventy looks like. Every time you remain independent at eighty, you inspire others to believe they can too.

Aging with capability is not just about you. It is about changing the narrative around aging for everyone who watches you. It is about proving that decline is not destiny. It is about showing that strength, vitality, and independence are available to those who practice.

Be the person who makes others rethink what aging means. Be the person who proves that seventy, eighty, and beyond can be strong, capable, and vibrant. Be the example that inspires change.

Wherever you are on the timeline, this message is for you.

If You Are in Your 30s:

You are building the foundation. The habits you establish now, the muscle you build now, the cardiovascular fitness you develop now—these are investments that will compound for decades.

You have time on your side. Use it. Don't wait until problems appear. Don't assume youth grants immunity from decline. Start now. Build capacity while it's still easy to build. Create a baseline of strength and fitness that will serve you for fifty years.

The work you do now prevents the crisis you will face later if you neglect it. Your future self is counting on you. Don't let them down.

If You Are in Your 40s:

You are at the inflection point. This is the decade when most people begin to notice changes. Energy drops. Weight creeps up. Recovery takes longer. Injuries appear.

These are not inevitable consequences of aging. These are warning signs that your current approach is not working. This is the moment to change course.

The good news: you still have time. Your body is still highly responsive to training and nutrition. You can reverse the early signs of decline. You can rebuild what has been lost. You can set a new trajectory.

But this is the decade where action matters most. Ignore the signals now, and the next decade becomes much harder. Respond to them now, and you redefine what the next thirty years look like.

If You Are in Your 50s:

You may have noticed significant changes. Muscle is harder to maintain. Fat is easier to gain. Sleep is less reliable. Joints ache more than they used to.

This is the decade that separates those who coast into decline from those who fight for capability. The choice is yours.

You cannot reverse time, but you can reverse much of the decline. Resistance training still builds muscle. Protein still supports recovery. Zone 2 cardio still improves metabolic health. Mobility work still enhances joint function.

It will take more effort than it would have ten years ago. It will require more patience, more consistency, and more attention to recovery. But it is possible. You can get stronger. You can feel better. You can regain capacity you thought was lost.

The only question is whether you will try. The effort is worth it. Your independence depends on it.

If You Are in Your 60s or Beyond:

You are the proof that age is not destiny. Every rep you complete, every walk you take, every meal you choose with intention—you are rewriting the script on aging.

You may be dealing with injuries, chronic conditions, or limitations that younger people don't face. This doesn't disqualify you. It means you need to adapt. Work with your doctor. Modify exercises as needed. Progress more slowly. But keep moving.

Strength training at your age is not optional. It is essential. Muscle mass is the difference between independence and dependence. Balance training is the difference between mobility and a fall that changes everything. Cardiovascular fitness is the difference between vitality and exhaustion.

You have lived long enough to see others decline. You have watched friends and family lose capability, lose independence, lose the ability to do the things they love. You know where that path leads.

You are choosing a different path. You are proving that decline is not inevitable. You are showing everyone around you what's possible.

Continue. Persist. Inspire. You are more important than you realize.

This book is not a blueprint for perfection. It is a guide for practice.

You will not execute every recipe perfectly. You will not complete every workout as prescribed. You will not sleep eight hours every night. You will not balance stress flawlessly. You will have setbacks, interruptions, and failures.

This is expected. This is normal. This is part of the process.

Longevity is not about perfection. It is about persistence. It is about showing up, even when you don't feel like it. It is about making the better choice, even when the worse choice is easier. It is about returning to the practice after you fall away from it.

The people who succeed are not the ones who never stumble. They are the ones who stumble and keep walking. They are the ones who miss a week and return the next. They are the ones who mess up and start again without self-judgment or shame.

You will mess up. When you do, forgive yourself. Learn from it if there's something to learn. Then return to the practice. Always return to the practice.

Over time, the practice becomes identity. The identity becomes life. And the life you build through consistent practice is one of strength, vitality, capability, and independence.

That life is not a gift. It is not luck. It is not genetics. It is a choice, made daily, over years and decades. It is the choice to train. The choice to eat well. The choice to recover. The choice to keep going when it would be easier to quit.

Make that choice today. Make it tomorrow. Make it ten thousand more times over the next fifty years.

That is how you outlive.

That is how you age with dignity, strength, and joy.

That is how you build a body and a life that lasts.

The practice begins now. And it never ends.

You now hold everything you need: the knowledge of how metabolism works, the recipes that support it, the training program that builds capacity, the recovery practices that enable adaptation, and the mindset that sustains it all.

But the book is complete only when you close it and begin.

Begin today. Begin imperfectly. Begin with one meal, one workout, one night of good sleep. Then do it again. And again. And again.

The compound interest of small actions, repeated over time, is the only true magic in health and fitness. There are no shortcuts. There are no hacks. There is only the practice.

Commit to the practice. Not for twelve weeks. Not for a year. For the rest of your life.

Your future self, strong and capable at eighty, will thank you for starting today.